JOHNS HOPKINS HEALTH

Back Pain

Johns Hopkins USA assists out-of-town patients with any aspect of arranging a visit to the Johns Hopkins Medical Institutions— from scheduling appointments to providing guidance on hotels, transportation, and preferred routes of travel. The program has up-to-date information on clinical practices and is a resource center for maps, visitor guides, and other materials of interest to non-local patients. Client Services Coordinators in the Johns Hopkins USA office are available Monday through Friday from 8:30 a.m. until 5:00 p.m. (Eastern). They can be reached toll-free at 1-800-507-9952 or locally at 410-614-USA1. You can also visit Johns Hopkins on the World Wide Web at *http://hopkins.med.jhu.edu/*.

JOHNS HOPKINS HEALTH

Back Pain:
What You
Need to Know

The information in this book is for your general knowledge only.
It is not intended as a substitute for the advice of a physician.
You should seek prompt medical care for any specific
medical problems you may have.

Published by Ottenheimer Publishers, Inc.
5 Park Center Court, Suite 300
Owings Mills, MD 21117-5001

Printed and bound in the United States of America

JH003M L K J I H G F E D C B A
ISBN 0-8241-0230-4

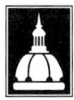

CONTENTS

INTRODUCTION

If you remember your high school biology lessons, a pivotal moment in human evolution took place when our ancestors dusted off their knuckles and started walking on two legs. With their hands freed from the burden of walking, they were able to use them for more useful things, such as making tools, planting crops, and a million or so years later, throwing baseballs and hauling groceries out of the car.

Walking upright may have been an evolutionary milestone, but it came with a price: Standing upright puts enormous pressure on the spine, especially in the lumbar (lower back) region. What's more, it requires that the spine be in nearly constant motion. Think about it: How many things can you do without bending or flexing your back? Every time you pick up a book, straighten your socks, or lift a laundry basket off the floor, your spine undergoes additional wear and tear.

Doctors estimate that 80 percent of Americans, about 200 million of us, will eventually have trouble with their lower backs. In fact, back pain is second only to the common cold as a reason for going to the doctor. Our backs may be versatile, but they're very prone to problems.

Unfortunately, we can't trade in our backs for new ones, although many people wish they could. If you have back problems you can be strong and fit one day and laid up with muscle spasms the next. You can bend over to tie your shoes and be unable to stand back up. Even watching too much television—sitting is very hard on the lower back—can land you in bed for a week.

The back, as with any other "machine," wears down over time. That's why back problems are relatively uncommon in young people but get increasingly common as we get older. The spinal disks can dry and crack, leading to herniated disks. The bony vertebrae get rough and weak and sometimes fracture. Even minor wear and tear on the spine can lead to inflammation, muscle spasms, and pain.

Back problems aren't merely uncomfortable. They're also slow to heal and quick to return. That's what makes back problems so discouraging—they can literally last your whole life. People with back pain are often anxious and worried. They lose time from their jobs, lose interest in sex, feel physically weak and tired. It's not surprising that doctors consider back problems to be among the most serious health concerns facing Americans today.

TAKING CHARGE

Back problems aren't always debilitating, of course. For most people, the pain is temporary and can be controlled with simple home remedies such as taking aspirin or ibuprofen, applying an ice pack or a heating pad, and not overdoing it for a few days.

What's more, there are many ways to prevent back pain from coming back—or even occurring in the first place. Most of these strategies are quite simple. Going for walks, stretching your muscles, and making slight changes in the ways you sit, stand, or pick up things will go a long way toward keeping your back healthy.

In this book we'll show you everything you need to do to keep your back strong. We'll begin by showing you how the back is designed—where it's weak and where it's strong—and what you can do to make it stronger. We'll also discuss the many ways in which a healthy lifestyle, such as eating well and getting regular exercise, can head off back pain. Most of the strategies are wonderfully simple—such as putting a pillow behind your back when you drive, for example, or using your legs more than your back when lifting heavy loads.

Since there's no guarantee of a life free of back pain, we'll show you how to take advantage of the best home treatments. We'll also guide you through the thicket of back-care options—everything from surgery and medical tests to alternative treatments such as chiropractic, massage, and even acupuncture. Most importantly, we'll help you understand which back problems can be treated at home and which demand professional care.

There's never a good time to have back problems, of course, but the treatment options available today are superb and getting better. Medical tests such as magnetic resonance imaging (MRI) can detect problems that were once impossible to find. Spinal surgery has advanced rapidly. In some cases it's even being done on an out-patient basis, without general anesthesia and long hospital stays.

One of the most exciting breakthroughs in recent years is a new way to treat fractured spinal vertebrae, a common cause of disability in older women. Doctors at The Johns Hopkins Medical Institutions, who are among the nation's leaders in back pain treatment and research, have pioneered a procedure in which it may be possible to actually glue fractured vertebrae back together—without surgery.

Doctors are very motivated to find new solutions to back pain (after all, they have back problems just as often as the rest of us), and many exciting developments are on the horizon. New drugs are being investigated for osteoporosis, the destructive bone condition that often leads to back pain. And research institutions such as Johns Hopkins are also examining the impact of emotions on back pain—everything from stress and anxiety to unhappiness on the job.

The Johns Hopkins University (including its world-renowned schools of medicine, nursing, and public health) and the closely related Johns Hopkins Health System are well-known for their commitment to medical research, education, and patient care. For the past seven years, The Johns Hopkins Hospital has been ranked the number one hospital in the United States in an annual survey conducted by *U. S. News and World Report*.

In this book Johns Hopkins presents a comprehensive, clearly written guide to the challenge of life with back pain. When it comes to health advice, you want expert knowledge and compassionate guidance, and that's precisely what you'll find here. The information in this book is based on the latest research and on years of experience of the finest health professionals anywhere. You can be assured that what you read within these pages is information you can trust, and just what you need at your side in your fight against back pain.

Why Does Your Back Hurt?

Back pain is an equal-opportunity annoyer. It forced Christine Todd Whitman, the governor of New Jersey, to take a week off from work. Football and baseball star Deion Sanders was temporarily sidelined with back-related pain and numbness in his leg. Joan Lunden of *Good Morning America* spent several days away from the camera because of problems with vertebrae in her neck. And basketball great Larry Bird retired from the Boston Celtics when he was 35 because of a bad back.

As millions of Americans can attest, it doesn't take much to throw the back out of whack. Swinging a golf club, putting groceries away, or simply letting loose with a good sneeze can sometimes result in days of excruciating pain.

Doctors estimate that eight out of 10 Americans will, at some time in their lives, have back pain. Sometimes the cause of the pain is serious—a herniated spinal disk, for example, or a fractured spinal vertebra. More often, back pain is caused by a temporary injury such as a muscle spasm or sprained ligament and will clear up on its own. But even "minor" back problems can cause major pain. What's more, people who have had one episode of back pain are very likely to have another. It's hard to live a normal life when you're worried that the next bout of pain may be just around the corner.

One of the most frustrating things about back pain is that it's almost impossible to predict. Sure, hauling boxes of books up the stairs can bring it on. But so can bending over to pick up the kids' clutter or sleeping in an awkward position. Even doctors are often frustrated by back pain because it's frequently hard to tell what's causing it. In fact, fewer than one in five cases of back pain can be specifically diagnosed by general means.

There are many underlying factors that can lead to back pain. We'll discuss the more common causes, as well as some that are rare but dangerous, in more detail in chapter 2. In the meantime, we'll take a look at the different types of back pain and who's most likely to get them. We'll also talk a bit about how your back is constructed, so you'll have a better idea of how it can go wrong—and what you can do to make it right.

On an encouraging note, keep in mind that the vast majority of back-pain episodes—about nine out of 10— will clear up on their own or with simple self-help measures. What's more, if you are one of those people who are prone to back pain, there are many things you can do to prevent it from coming back.

ACUTE AND CHRONIC BACK PAIN

Back pain can be sharp or dull, constant or intermittent. A backache can come on suddenly or gradually. And despite the name, back problems don't affect only the back. People with a herniated spinal disk, for example, will not only have a sore back, but possibly pain or numbness in the buttocks, legs, or feet.

Doctors divide back pain into two main categories, acute or chronic, depending on how long the pain lasts.

Acute Back Pain

Acute back pain is pain that comes on suddenly. Often caused by injury to a muscle or ligament, acute pain is short-lived, lasting from a few days to a few weeks.

Acute back pain, which is most common in adults under 60, often responds well to home treatments. Doctors usually advise people with acute pain to take it easy for a few days and to use over-the-counter (and sometimes prescription) medications such as aspirin or ibuprofen to control pain and inflammation. Applying cold or hot packs is also helpful for relieving pain and muscle spasms.

Acute back pain may not stick around long, but it often comes back. In fact, if you've had one episode, you have a 50-50 chance of having another within the next two years. To reduce the risk, doctors usually advise people to begin a gradual stretching and strengthening program. It's also important to learn to use your back in ways that will help keep it strong and healthy. (You'll read more about biome-chanics—the science of proper ways to use your body—in chapter 6.)

Chronic Back Pain

The human back isn't really designed to withstand a lifetime of bending, getting in and out of cars, and hauling heavy objects. Over time, the spinal disks and vertebrae that make up the spine gradually begin to wear. In fact, the spine is the first functional unit in the human body to begin to wear out. This can result in nagging backaches that seem to last forever. This type of pain is called chronic, which doctors define as lasting longer than 12 weeks.

Chronic back pain, which is often (but not always) more serious than the acute kind, may be caused by fractured ver-tebrae, a herniated spinal disk, spinal stenosis (a narrowing of the spinal canal), and various forms of arthritis. Chronic back pain appears especially often in older people, although the most common cause isn't really aging itself—it's simply "wear and tear."

Chronic back problems are generally less painful than those that are accompanied by sudden, acute pain. But their stubborn persistence is emotionally and physically draining. Constant pain makes people frustrated, tired, and irritable. It's hard to sleep when your back hurts, and it's hard to stay active—an essential part of most back-recovery plans—when you're tired all the time.

Because it lasts so long, chronic pain can have a devastating impact on your emotional, social, and even financial well-being. It can affect your job, your friends, and your family. Many sufferers of chronic pain refrain from sexual intimacy with their spouses because they're afraid that sex will be painful or cause even more damage. This can put a strain on any relationship.

Chronic back pain is often treated in the same ways as the acute kind, at least at first. But because the conditions that cause chronic pain are often serious, home remedies such as rest and over-the-counter medications aren't always effective. Nonetheless, one of the most powerful "remedies" is still within your control. To avoid the downward cycle of pain and depression, it's essential to keep your spirits up. That's not always easy to do, of course, but it can play an important role in helping you recover more quickly.

SCIATICA: THE PAIN OF INJURED NERVES

One type of acute or chronic back pain, and one of the most severe, is caused by a condition called sciatica. Caused by pressure on nerves (the sciatic nerves), sciatica can send shooting pains down the buttocks into one or both legs below the knee. The pain may be accompanied by weakness, numbness, or an uncomfortable pins-and-needles sensation.

The sciatic nerves are located in the lower part of the spine and extend down the buttocks and the back of each leg. Anything that presses against one or both of these nerves is going to cause excruciating pain. People with a herniated disk, for example, often get shooting pains down one leg when portions of the damaged disk press against the nerve. Spinal stenosis, in which the spinal canal or other portions of the spine get narrower, can be even more serious. It typically puts pressure on both of the lumbar nerve roots, sending pain down both legs.

People with sciatica often find that lying flat on their back with their knees slightly raised is the only position that makes the pain go away, at least some of the time. Other positions—bending over to retrieve something you've dropped, for example—can be exceptionally painful.

WHO GETS BACK PAIN?

Back problems are influenced by heredity, your lifestyle, and your job. If your parents had back problems, you have a higher risk of getting them yourself. People whose jobs involve a lot of sitting, such as truck drivers, writers, or computer operators, have a very high risk of back pain because sitting is extremely hard on the back.

Not surprisingly, people who do a lot of lifting, such as nurses, also tend to have back problems. But here's a contributing factor that is surprising. Smoking is a very common cause of—or at least a major contributor to—back pain. Smoking reduces the amount of oxygen-rich blood that reaches parts of the back, which can cause the disks to break down more quickly. Being overweight can also be a problem because it puts additional strain on an already-overworked back. Even stress plays a role because it causes your muscles to be more tense and more likely to go into spasm. What's more, stress makes any symptom you already have seem all the more painful.

Back Pain and Age

Back pain is most common in people 30 to 60 years of age. That's when we're most active, and it's also the stage of life when the cumulative effects of aging are beginning to take their toll. As with any mechanical structure, the back naturally gets a bit weaker with age. In fact, among people 45 to 64, back pain trails only heart disease and arthritis as a cause for limiting daily activities. And while young people tend to recover quite quickly from back pain, the body's ability to heal itself does slow with age. As a result, older people with back pain often hurt more, and longer, than young folks do.

Every passing year, your back undergoes a number of changes that make it more susceptible to problems. Your stomach muscles gradually get weaker, providing less support for the lower back. And many of us let our belts out a notch or two as we get older, which gives the back more weight to carry around. Plus, a lifetime of bending, twisting, and simply standing upright causes wear and tear on the vertebrae, disks, and joints, which can lead to painful problems.

Once we reach 50, the major causes of back pain are degenerative—that is, they're caused by gradual wear and tear on the spine. The most common degenerative condition affecting the spine is wear of the disks, which causes altered motion. And that in turn results in worn-out spinal joints. Other common causes are spinal stenosis, vertebral compression fractures, and herniated disks.

In younger folks, of course, wear and tear is less of an issue. However, they're the ones most likely to be participating in vigorous activities, such as sports, dancing, and exercise. That's why they're most at risk for sudden back injuries, including strains, sprains, and herniated spinal disks.

Back Pain and Gender

Men and women suffer from back problems at about equal rates. The causes of the pain, however, are usually quite different.

Men, especially younger men, have traditionally been more physically active than women (in this culture, at any rate). They're more likely to be doing heavy lifting or long-distance driving, or playing rough-and-tumble team sports. As a result, they're more at risk for sudden, traumatic injuries that cause back pain, such as herniated disks and spinal fractures. As men get older and less active, however, their risk of back problems actually becomes lower than women's.

Women face different kinds of concerns. Young women have a fairly low risk of back problems. One exception to this rule, as every Mom-to-be knows, is pregnancy. The weight of the baby puts a lot of strain on the lower back. To make things worse, all of that weight is concentrated in one small bundle of joy, pushing the center of gravity forward and putting additional pressure on the lower back. What's more, as a woman approaches delivery, the body releases hormones that relax the muscles in preparation for giving birth. This is very handy for labor, but not so good for the back.

Older women have different back concerns. After menopause, when a woman's estrogen levels begin to decline, her bones may become thinner and weaker. This condition, caused osteoporosis, makes many women particularly vulnerable to spinal fractures known as vertebral compression fractures. (Older men also get these fractures, but less than half as frequently as women do.)

Doctors estimate that 25 percent of American women over age 50 will experience painful compression fractures of the vertebrae at some time in their lives. (For information on preventing osteoporosis, see pages 47 and 121.)

Back Pain and Your Job

Not surprisingly, people who spend their days doing heavy lifting, such as warehouse or construction workers, often have problems with back pain. In fact, back pain was a major problem at Home Depot stores in California—so much so that the company implemented a strategy in which many employees were required to wear back-supporting belts or braces. (To learn more about Home Depot's new policy—and its surprising aftermath—see page 102.)

It's not just heavy lifting that causes problems on the job. Office workers will often have back problems because

---

THE RISK FACTORS

There are hundreds, if not thousands, of things that can cause back pain. Some of the most common risk factors include:

- Age 30 to 60 years
- Sedentary occupation or lifestyle
- Long-distance driving
- Frequent bending or twisting
- Participation in sports such as gymnastics, golf, diving, weight-lifting, tennis, or football
- Obesity
- Depression, stress, or anxiety
- Dissatisfaction with work
- Smoking
- Poor posture
- Heavy lifting

sitting puts a tremendous amount of pressure on the spinal disks. Long-distance driving is even worse. Not only are you sitting for long periods of time, but vibrations in the car or truck can accelerate the rate at which the spinal disks and vertebrae break down.

Studies have also shown that psychological factors at work play a major role in back problems. People who are depressed or unhappy with their jobs often complain of back problems. That makes sense because stress and anxiety cause muscle tension, and tense muscles are more prone to injuries. What's more, people who are stressed respond to pain differently than those who aren't. They hurt more.

HOW YOUR BACK WORKS

Your back is remarkably complex. It's strong, yet flexible. It's capable of bending forward, backward, and sideways. It permits ballet dancers to leap and spin, gymnasts to do handsprings off a narrow rail, and parents to lift their toddlers off the floor.

The same complexity that makes the back so versatile, however, also makes it vulnerable. The spine consists of dozens of interrelated parts—not just bones but also muscles, ligaments, joints, and disks. When something goes wrong with any one of these parts, the entire back may be affected.

In the following pages we'll take a look at the design of the spine and how the different parts work together to form a solid, but not always trouble-free, whole. It's a short but simple course in back anatomy, and it'll be worth your while. When you get to know all the parts of your back, you'll be better equipped to take advantage of new strategies against the pain.

ANATOMY OF THE SPINE

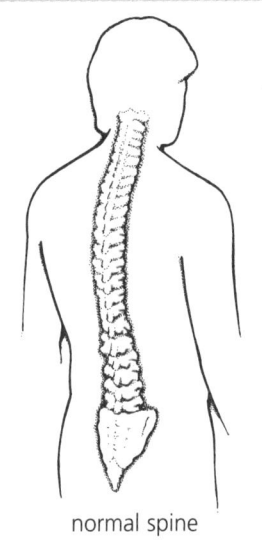

normal spine

Your spine is a remarkable piece of engineering. Even though it consists of 24 individual bones—the vertebrae—and is in nearly constant motion, it is strong enough to hold you upright and mobile enough so you can bend and twist. At the same time, it protects the spinal cord within a hard, bony shell.

The spine gains much of its stability from the way the vertebrae are locked together. Each vertebra has seven bony, spike-like protrusions called processes. Four of these processes lock into their mates on adjoining vertebrae. (The other three are used to anchor muscles to the spine.) The place where the bones lock together is called a facet joint. These joints keep the vertebrae stable while at the same time allowing them to shift and move when you do.

The smallest vertebrae are in the neck. Called cervical vertebrae, they support the head and are designed more for mobility than strength. Lower down are the thoracic vertebrae, which support the weight of your arms and trunk. Lower still, in the lower back, are the lumbar vertebrae. These are the sturdiest of the vertebrae, since it's their job to support the entire weight of your body. At the very bottom of the spine are nine vertebrae that have become fused together. They make up the sacrum (the back of the pelvis) and the coccyx (the tailbone.)

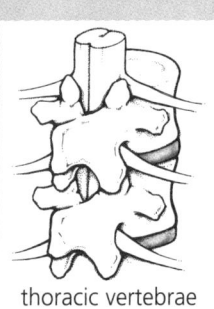

thoracic vertebrae

Your vertebrae don't sit directly on top of each other. Between them is a tough, gel-filled disk that resembles a jelly doughnut. These disks, called spinal disks, help absorb the shocks when you walk, sit down, or pick up a paper clip.

The vertebrae themselves are not solid bone. At the rear of each vertebra is a hole. When the vertebrae are stacked one on top of the other, these holes line up, forming the spinal canal. This canal is what protects the spinal nerves. Nerves that branch off from the spine are also protected—not by the spinal canal, but by bony passages in the vertebrae.

The Vertebrae

We often think of the spine as a single unit, but in fact it's a veritable jigsaw puzzle of 24 interlocking bones called vertebrae. Each vertebra joins the next at a slight angle, forming a graceful S-shaped curve that supports the weight of your body. The curve provides stability and allows your spine to absorb shocks and stresses. In addition, the bony vertebrae form a tough shell, protecting your spinal cord and the nerves inside.

The vertebrae themselves can be divided into different parts. In your neck, for example, there are seven small, flexible vertebrae (the cervical vertebrae), which allow you to turn your head. Lower down in the chest area are the 12, slightly larger thoracic vertebrae, which support the weight of your arms and trunk. The remaining five vertebrae (the lumbar vertebrae) are the largest and strongest. Located in the lower back, they help support the weight of your entire body.

It makes sense that vertebrae get progressively larger toward the bottom. The lower vertebrae act like the foundation of a house, carrying the heaviest load. Those at the top, on the other hand, are designed more for flexibility than for bearing weight.

You may think of your vertebrae as though each is a solid, simple unit, but their construction is really more complex than that. Each vertebra consists of an oval-shaped bone that is studded with seven bony projections called spinal processes. Four of these projections, which jut out from the rear of the vertebrae, interlock with their counterparts on adjacent vertebrae. They help lock your vertebrae together, just like the pieces of a jigsaw puzzle.

The places where these bony projections mesh are called facet joints. Tough bands of fibrous ligaments lock each facet joint to the next. Some of the bony projections act as anchor points for muscles, which give your back strength and stability. Together, the vertebrae, ligaments, and muscles of the back and abdomen are what hold you upright.

The vertebrae themselves are simply the bony part of the spine. Surrounding each vertebra is a layer—a cushion, you might say—of fat, blood, and other body fluids. Doctors refer to the whole package—the vertebra plus the surrounding material—as the vertebral motion segment.

At the base of the spine where the vertebrae end is a triangular piece of bone called the sacrum. (The sacrum actually consists of vertebrae, but because they're all fused together they're considered one unit.) At the bottom of the sacrum is a bone called the coccyx (tailbone). Together, the sacrum and the coccyx join the pelvic bones at either side to form a solid base. This base is what supports your entire spine.

The Spinal Disks

If you've ever had back problems or know someone who has, you've heard the expression "slipped disk." But what, exactly, is a disk?

Spinal vertebrae don't sit directly on top of each other. Between each one is a pad of cartilage called an intervertebral disk—or just disk, for short. These disks, which make up a third of the length of your spine, act as cushions and shock absorbers. They prevent the bony vertebrae from grinding against each other as you move around.

Your disks aren't hard, lifeless little pads. They're living tissue that's constantly moving, expanding, and contracting to accommodate the moving vertebrae they support.

Each disk has an inner and outer part. The outer part, called the annulus fibrosus, is made up of many overlapping layers of collagen—a tough tissue that expands and contracts and moves when you do, much as a radial tire on your car does when it meets the changing surface of the road.

Within this tough covering is a soft, jelly-like center called the nucleus pulposus. This inner portion of the disk contains a lot of water. The water is under pressure so it's constantly pushing outward against the outer portion of the disk. The pressure keeps the disk taut so it is always in firm contact with the vertebrae above and below. In addition, the fluid nature of the center adds elasticity to the disk, allowing it to change shape to accommodate the shifting vertebrae.

Disks don't necessarily last forever. Like shock absorbers on your car, they wear out and lose their "give." This usually happens because the soft, inner portion dries and shrinks over time. As it loses moisture and flexibility, it also loses its ability to cushion and protect the vertebrae. And as disks dry out, they lose height, which is why we all grow a little shorter as we age.

The outer part of the disk can also become less flexible. By the time we've reached middle age, cracks will sometimes appear in the thick outer layer of a disk. If the crack is large enough, the soft material inside the disk may bulge out, like the filling of a jelly doughnut. Doctors call this a herniated or "slipped" disk.

A herniated disk isn't always painful. In fact, many people with herniated disks don't even know they have them. If the bulging material happens to press against the sciatic nerve, however, you're likely to know there's a problem. Of all the problems affecting the back, the pain from sciatica is among the most severe.

The Ligaments

Spinal ligaments are sturdy bands of fibrous tissue that run the length of the spine. Stretchy and strong, they're responsible for holding your vertebrae and disks in place.

The major spinal ligaments are the most elastic parts of your body, but they gradually lose their stretch over time. This creates additional pressure inside the spinal disks, which can cause them to wear, leaving the vertebrae to rub against each other in ways nature didn't intend. This abnormal movement can also cause the vertebrae to form bony projections called bone spurs. These are "degenerative" arthritic changes. In other words, the vertebrae get larger, which in turn can cause spinal stenosis, a narrowing of the passages within the spine.

The Joints

We've seen how the spine's facet joints hold vertebrae together while allowing the spine to move and flex. Like any joint in the body, the facet joints will occasionally undergo arthritic changes such as swelling and stiffness, causing pain in the back.

One joint in particular, the sacroiliac joint (where the bottom of the spine meets the pelvis), is vulnerable to a less common type of arthritis called ankylosing spondylitis. We'll discuss this in more detail in chapter 2. For now we'll just say that this condition can cause the joint to become

MUSCLES THAT SUPPORT THE BACK

The human back is not only strong, but remarkably limber. There's a good reason for this. Surrounding the spine are 140 layers of overlapping muscles. These muscles are what permit your back and spine to move—forward, backward, and sideways, as well as when you twist. Of course, these are also the muscles that hurt when you spend too much time in the garden or slip on an icy step.

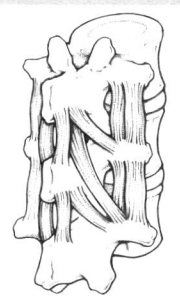

short muscles

Each of these muscles does a different job. Deep in the back near the spine are three groups of short muscles. One group is made up of the intertransverse muscles, which allow you to bend sideways. Another group consists of the interspinal muscles, which let you bend backward. Finally, there are the rotator muscles, which help you to move from side to side.

Farther out from the spine are two larger muscles. Called the erector spinae, these muscles extend down either side of the lower back. Their jobs are to help you move, to support the spine and to absorb the stresses that occur every time you move your back.

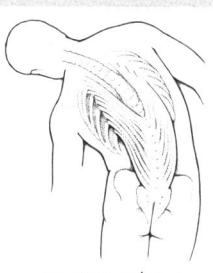

erector spinae

Finally, there's an outer layer of muscles that is clearly visible from the outside of the upper back. These muscles are the trapezius and the latissimus dorsi. Their primary job is to move your shoulders and arms, although they help your back move, too.

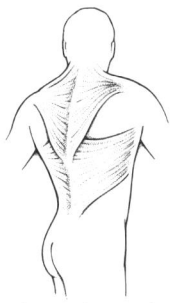

trapezius and
latissimus dorsi

swollen and inflamed, sometimes causing excruciating pain to flare up in your back.

The Muscles

Surrounding your spine are 140 layers of overlapping muscles that provide support and strength. As with any muscle, they can get strained or stretched, and when this happens they can lock down into painful spasms.

Deep in the back are three muscle groups that, along with ligaments, help hold the vertebrae together. One muscle group, the intertransverse muscles, allows you to bend sideways. Another group, the interspinal muscles, lets you bend backward. The third group, the rotator muscles, enables you to twist from side to side.

Nearer the surface are two larger muscles called the erector spinae. These muscles run down either side of your lower back. They not only help you move, but they also support the spine and absorb stress. These muscles are the ones most likely to go into painful spasms.

Another key back muscle is the psoas muscle, which extends across the hip joint and attaches to the thighbone. This muscle sometimes gets strained when people do sit-ups the old-fashioned way—by keeping their legs straight out instead of slightly bent.

Two large muscles in the upper back, the trapezius and the latissimus dorsi, are mainly responsible for moving your shoulders and arms. They also assist in back movement. Finally, there are your abdominal muscles, or "abs," which link together with the back muscles to support the spine.

The Spinal Cord and Nerves

We couldn't live without the spinal cord—which is why it's well protected within nearly solid bone. It is responsible for carrying messages between the brain and the rest of the body.

Each vertebra has a hole toward the back. With the vertebrae stacked one on top of the other, these holes line up to form the spinal canal, which in turn contains the spinal cord.

Like an electrical cable inside your house, your spinal cord doesn't work alone. All along its length are complex bundles of nerve branches, which exit the spinal cord and snake between hollow spaces in the vertebrae called foramina. These nerves then leave the spinal area and travel to all the parts of your body.

Even though most of your spinal cord is well protected, one part is out in the open. At about waist-level the spinal cord ends its journey. It emerges from the bony protection of the spine, forming a thick bundle of nerves called the cauda equina, or horse's tail. The nerves in this bundle are each targeted to specific muscles that control your legs, bladder, bowels, sexual organs, and spinal disks.

It doesn't happen often, but sometimes a piece of bone will press against the cauda equina. This can result in numbness, loss of bowel or bladder control, or other serious symptoms. Pressure on the cauda equina is always considered an emergency, and surgery will usually be scheduled right away.

The Weakest Link

It's really not surprising that when people talk about back pain they're usually referring to pain in the lower back, since it's the lower (or lumbar) part of the spine that carries the heaviest load.

Just how vulnerable is your lower back? Doctors agree that low-back pain is one of the biggest causes of disability,

---

**ANATOMY OF THE SPINE:
THE SHORT VERSION**

Your spine is an incredibly complex piece of engineering.
Here's what it contains:

- *Vertebrae.* A stack of 24 interlocking bones that form an S-shaped curve.
- *Disks.* Cushions between the vertebrae that stabilize and protect the spine.
- *Ligaments.* Tough bands that hold disks and vertebrae in place.
- *Joints.* The place where muscles, ligaments, and bones come together. The joints allow movement and flexibility.
- *Muscles.* They control movement and give strength and stability to the spine.
- *Spinal Cord and Nerves.* They carry electrical signals throughout the body.

---

not only in the United States but in many other parts of the world, as well.

Putting It All Together

When you consider all the parts that make up your back—the vertebrae, disks, ligaments, joints, and muscles—the amazing thing isn't that we have back problems but that we don't have them more often. The fact that most of us experience only occasional trouble proves that the basic construction of the spine is very solid indeed.

In a way, the one flaw in the system is its very complexity. Everything is packed very closely together—muscles, joints, bones and, more importantly, the nerves. What this means is that any time something goes wrong—a disk ruptures, a muscle goes into spasm, or a joint gets inflamed—

there's probably a nearby nerve that's going to get irritated and inflamed. This is why even minor back problems can often cause serious pain.

THE IMPACT OF BACK PAIN

You would think back pain might be most common in parts of the world where most people make their living through hard physical labor. But in fact, back pain appears to be most common in "advanced," industrialized countries.

We work at desks instead of in the fields, and drive cars instead of walking. As we've seen, sitting puts enormous pressure on the spinal disks—much more than walking does—and driving is even worse. We don't always get a lot of exercise, either, which means our muscles aren't always able to give our spines the support they need.

And consider our high-speed, nine-to-five lives, and hurried lunch hours spent rushing through fast-food lines. It's easy for us to take in too many calories and hard to take off the pounds. No wonder back pain in this country has reached nearly epidemic proportions.

The costs of back pain—to you when you're hurting and to society as a whole—are enormous. For example:

- Every year, one in four people will stay home from work because of back pain, making it the leading cause of absenteeism in the workplace.
- Nationally, the medical cost of treating back pain— which is the second most common reason people see their doctors—is about $25 billion a year.
- The average medical bill for people needing surgery for back pain is almost $14,000.
- The total cost of back pain, including health care, days lost from work, and lost productivity, is thought to be $80 to $100 billion a year.

The real cost of back pain, of course, is to the unfortunate person who wakes up one morning unable to get out of bed. Who can't lift her toddler without getting down on her knees. Who finds himself turning down invitations because standing at a social gathering is simply too painful. And dancing's out of the question.

But there's no reason to be at the mercy of your back pain. In the following chapter we'll look further at the causes and symptoms of back pain, and also at what you can do to keep it under control.

Symptoms and Causes of Back Pain

Back pain is so common and occurs so frequently that you'd think doctors would have it pretty well mapped out by now. Within five minutes of walking into your doctor's office, you'd have all the answers: what the problem is, what caused it, and what you need to do to fix it.

Most of the time, however, all that can be said for certain is that you hurt. What's actually causing the problem often remains a mystery. There are several reasons for this. For one thing, back pain is often caused by soft tissue injuries— sprained muscles, for example—which don't readily reveal themselves on X-rays or through other standard medical tests.

In addition, back pain doesn't always appear where the actual injury is. It's not uncommon, for example, for people to have herniated disks in their backs while the pain occurs in their buttocks or legs. It's often hard to know exactly where the trouble got started.

What's more, back pain can't always be linked to a specific accident or situation. When you get a black eye, you know exactly what caused it (and you'll surely remember to close that closet door in the future). Back pain, however, often appears to come out of nowhere. It may be caused by old injuries that never healed properly, or by gradual wear and tear on your spinal joints or disks. In fact, it's not uncommon for people to develop back problems after letting loose with a hearty sneeze. You know the sneeze didn't really cause the problem, but what did?

MAKING A DIAGNOSIS

Doctors are able to pinpoint the cause of back pain by routine means in fewer than one in five cases. That sounds serious, but fortunately, it usually doesn't matter all that much. Doctors have a lot of experience handling back pain. They can help you feel better and suggest ways to prevent future problems even when they don't know exactly what's causing the pain.

In any event, the truly mysterious kinds of back pain—the cases that have doctors and patients scratching their heads—most often clear up on their own or with simple home care. By contrast, the types of back problems that are potentially serious, such as infections, tumors, spinal stenosis (a narrowing around the spinal cord or spinal roots), and herniated disks, are easily detected with standard medical tests. The diagnosis is generally easy.

Regardless of the type of back pain you have, you can help your doctor make an accurate diagnosis by keeping notes of your symptoms or even by keeping a "back pain diary." Don't walk into your doctor's office and simply say "It hurts." Your doctor will want to know where you hurt. Is the pain in your lower back or a little higher up? Is it in your legs? Is it constant, or does it come and go? The more information you can give, the more effective—and possibly less expensive—your treatment is likely to be.

Don't wait too long to see your doctor, either. It's normal for backaches to last a few days. But if the pain is severe or lasting longer than you think it should, it's time to pick up the phone. This is especially true if you have other symptoms along with the pain, such as a loss of bowel or bladder control or tingling or numbness in one or both of your legs. (See "Serious Warning Signs" in chapter 3 for more details on severe symptoms and when to seek medical help.)

THE CAUSES OF BACK PAIN

Except in the case of sudden injury—from a car accident, for example—back problems rarely develop overnight. Even when the pain comes on suddenly, you can bet that the underlying problem was months or years in the making.

To a certain extent, time is your back's worst enemy. Years of hauling groceries, tying your shoes, playing tennis, or simply sitting on the couch and watching television can gradually weaken the back, making it more susceptible to injuries or wear-and-tear conditions such as osteoarthritis.

In addition, many of the things we do every day can have a direct impact on the health of our backs. People with poor posture, for example, often lose strength in certain muscles, which deprives the back of essential support. Back problems can also arise from lifestyle issues. People who don't exercise and spend a lot of time sitting, for example, have a high risk of herniated spinal disks. Being overweight often contributes to back problems. So do smoking cigarettes and experiencing a lot of stress. Even spending a lot of the time in the car may cause the spine to weaken and eventually break down.

In young people, most flare-ups of back pain are caused by "pulling" a muscle or ligament, or by small tears in the outer portion of the disk. Most of the time, these are minor problems that usually clear up in a few days. As we get older, however, the causes of back pain tend to get more serious, and the pain has a way of sticking around longer. It's unfortunate, but the spine naturally deteriorates to some degree over time. Cartilage and vertebrae show signs of wear. Joints get looser and less secure in their movements. Each of these various factors can lead to swelling and inflammation, which in turn can cause long-lasting back pain.

Some of the most common long-term changes to the spine include herniated disks, fractures of the vertebrae, arthritis, and spondylolisthesis. We'll discuss each of these problems later. But the important thing to remember is this: Even though these conditions are caused to a certain extent by "natural" wear and tear on the spine, they aren't inevitable. There are many things you can do to minimize or even prevent the damage.

Occasionally, back pain is also caused by serious and hard-to-treat conditions, such as osteomyelitis (a spinal infection), cauda equina syndrome (a nerve disorder), and some kinds of cancer. Fortunately, most of these conditions are quite rare.

In the following pages, we'll take a look at the most common—and a few not-so-common—causes of back pain. We'll discuss the symptoms you need to watch for. More importantly, we'll show you a few ways to ease the discomfort and help prevent problems from occurring in the future. (For an in-depth look at treatments for back pain, see chapter 4.)

SPRAINS, STRAINS, AND SPASMS

We often use the terms "sprain" and "strain" interchangeably, but they actually refer to entirely different things. A sprain occurs when a ligament has been partly torn, while a strain means that you've pulled or overstretched a muscle.

What sprains and strains have in common is that they weaken the supporting structures (the muscles and ligaments) of the spine, making you more susceptible to further injuries—possibly more serious ones. What's more, both strains and sprains may result in muscle spasms, the painful contractions that are the muscle's way of telling you that it doesn't want to move anymore.

Sprained Ligaments

You can think of ligaments as tough rubber bands that connect muscles to bones—in this case, your vertebral bones. Ligaments help support and stabilize the vertebrae, while at the same time providing just enough flex for your spine to move when you do.

When you sprain a ligament, you've actually either torn or stretched it. Ligaments normally are pretty tough. Over time, however, they lose some of their elasticity. Like a rubber band that has been stretched a lot, they become looser and have less "give," making them more likely to sprain. And the outer covering of a disk, called the annulus, is actually a series of interwoven ligaments that can become torn. This is probably the most common cause of back pain.

Sprains usually occur when you've stretched a ligament farther than it wants to go or torn it—by hefting a heavy load, for example, or putting too much oomph into your golf swing. Even bending over to pick up a book can cause a painful sprain if your ligaments aren't as strong and flexible as they should be.

Strained Muscles

You use your back in almost everything you do, from lifting a coffee cup to getting up from your chair. To handle the load, your back is packed with muscles—140 altogether—which hold the spine straight and allow you to bend and twist.

When one or more of these muscles is overworked or out of shape, it can stretch beyond its normal range of motion. Doctors call this a muscle strain.

Strained muscles are common in young people, for the simple reason that they often push their bodies harder and farther than they were meant to go. And strains are also especially common in "weekend athletes"—folks who don't normally get regular exercise but decide to go all out at the company's annual volleyball game.

Like the engine in your car, your muscles need a little time to warm up before you put them in high gear. People who don't take the time to stretch or warm up will often spend the rest of the afternoon in bed wondering what they did to themselves.

Falls are another common cause of strained muscles. If you slip while walking across an icy parking lot to your car, you'll instinctively twist your body to keep your balance and stay on your feet. In the process of twisting, however, you may push a muscle beyond its normal limits.

There's no way to tell if you've strained a muscle or sprained a ligament. Your doctor may not be able to tell, either. But it doesn't really matter—they both hurt about the same!

Muscle Spasms

When you hurt your back—by straining a muscle, for example, or by rupturing a spinal disk—your muscles know that something is wrong. To protect themselves from further damage, muscles will sometimes contract into tough, painful little knots known as spasms. Muscle spasms prevent the muscles from moving, giving them a little breathing space in which to recover.

Spasms work, but at a cost—they can be extraordinarily painful. If you've ever had a charley horse, you know just how painful muscle spasms can be.

Spasms may occur at the instant of injury or hours or days later. Even if it has been years since an injury, the surrounding muscles may be just a little bit weak. The slightest "insult"—raking the yard, for example—can cause them to go into spasm. In fact, it's very common for muscle spasms to occur during simple, everyday activities such as putting groceries away or even climbing out of your car.

You can have muscle spasms even when you haven't hurt yourself at all—at least not in any obvious way. But your muscles know things you don't. When they're feeling tired or vulnerable, they may play it safe and lock into spasms. This is especially true of the erector spinae, the sensitive muscles in your lower back. They're the ones most likely to spasm.

Coping with Sprains, Strains, and Spasms

As we mentioned earlier, a strained muscle doesn't show up on X-rays. Even swelling and inflammation around the ligaments may be impossible to detect. But this doesn't really matter. Just as you can enjoy *60 Minutes* without understanding how your TV works, you can get relief from back pain even when the cause remains mysterious.

Back sprains and strains respond well to the same home remedies you'd use for any muscle problem: applying cold (such as an ice pack or a large bag of frozen peas) the first day to stop the swelling and relieve the pain, and using hot baths or hot pads after that to increase blood flow, speed healing, and reduce pain and spasm. Taking it easy for a few days will give your damaged muscles or ligaments time to heal. Aspirin or another over-the-counter pain reliever may also help.

When the pain is unusually severe, your doctor may prescribe muscle relaxants, which will help the muscles in spasm loosen their grip. Wearing a brace and getting a massage can also be helpful.

The problem with back pain, of course, is that it almost always comes back. Some people simply have a tendency to develop back problems. Others have lifestyles that involve plenty of vigorous activity—anything from working in the garden all day to playing soccer on weekends—which can put a lot of strain on the back. And in young people, back muscles support up to one-third of the load they carry.

By staying aware of your back and taking simple precautions—warming up before you exercise, for example, or using your legs more than your back when you lift—you can prevent a lot of strains and sprains from occurring in the first place.

In addition, exercise is an essential—though often overlooked—part of any back protection plan. The muscles in your back and abdomen need to be strong simply to withstand the daily effort of holding you upright. Abdominal exercises such as crunches are an excellent way to give strength and stability to your lower back. And the back muscles themselves, of course, also benefit from your working out. Your doctor, a physical therapist, or an athletic trainer will gladly recommend an exercise program that's best for you. Even if you have no intention of joining a gym or health club, simply walking, biking, or swimming will keep your muscles strong and out of trouble. (For more on using exercise to ease back pain, see chapter 7.)

DEGENERATIVE CHANGES

Given enough time, most everything wears out. That's true for the soles on your shoes and the engine in your car, and it's true for your back. After years of bending, twisting, and shifting back and forth, the bones that make up the spine get a little rough around the edges. Doctors refer to these changes as degenerative, or simply wear and tear.

Even though you're not usually aware of them, degenerative changes begin long before you pick up your first pair of bifocals. In fact, these changes usually begin around age 20 and sometimes even earlier. Doctors using a test called magnetic resonance imaging (MRI) have detected disk changes in teenagers, and the disks continue to lose fluid and shrink over the years.

It's hard to say anything good about degenerative changes to the spine, but there is one upside. By the time you reach age 60, the disks have lost so much fluid and flexibility that they're less likely to herniate (rupture) than when you were younger. On the other hand, increasingly rigid disks provide less protection to the bones of the spine, which allows other degenerative changes to occur.

The disks in the lumbar (lower back) region are often the first to go because they support the greatest load. In fact, pressure on the lumbar spine can be as much as 11 times your body weight, depending on what you're doing and your posture while you're doing it.

As the disks get harder and flatter—or, in some cases, wear away entirely—the vertebrae begin to rub and grind against each other. We don't usually think of bones as forming scar tissue, but in a sense they do. After years of grinding, the vertebrae sometimes develop bony spurs called osteophytes. In themselves, osteophytes don't hurt. But sometimes this extra bone presses against nearby nerves, which can be very painful.

Finally, your muscles naturally grow weaker with age. This contributes to degenerative changes because more stress falls on the spinal disks and facet joints. The facet joints themselves may also deteriorate over time, leading to pain and inflammation.

Degenerative changes occur throughout our bodies, of course. But those affecting the spine can be especially troublesome, if only because we depend on our backs for so many of our daily activities. As the spine becomes stiffer and less mobile, we notice it right away. It gets harder to hop out of bed in the morning or to lace a pair of shoes. In many families, the expression "Oh, my aching back" is heard almost as often as "Honey, would you get me another cup of coffee?"

Why We Lose Inches as We Gain Years

If you've watched your parents age (or you're getting up there yourself), you've probably noticed some changes in the height department. It's not your imagination: People really do get shorter as they get older. Here's why.

+ As muscles in the back and abdomen weaken, people have a natural tendency to stoop a bit.
+ The spinal disks get harder and flatter, "lowering" the spine.

DEGENERATIVE CHANGES AND SPINAL STENOSIS

Like the soles on your shoes or the engine in your car, your back naturally shows signs of wear over time. A lifetime of bending, walking, and dancing causes the various parts of the back—the vertebrae as well as the spinal disks—to crack, weaken, or simply wear away. Doctors refer to these effects as degenerative changes.

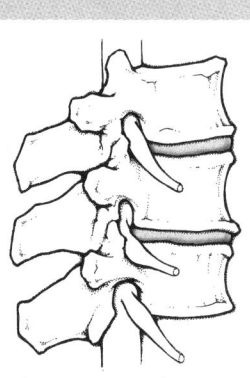
degenerative changes

There are many types of degenerative changes. The spinal disks can be especially hard hit. As you get older, the disks lose moisture, causing them to get flat and hard. This in turn makes them less able to cushion the spine—and more likely to rupture (or herniate).

Another degenerative change happens when the cartilage lining the facet joints—the joints that lock vertebrae together—wears

- Individual vertebrae sometimes collapse, thus further shortening the spine.

These changes are common and to a certain extent inevitable, but you can reduce "shrinkage" simply by keeping your muscles strong. Doing regular weight-bearing exercise—this can be as mundane as walking or as exciting as dancing—helps the muscles in your back hold you upright. What's more, regular exercise can actually help restore bone mass. In the following pages, we'll look at some of the more common wear-and-tear conditions that affect the spine, along with practical strategies for keeping your back strong and mobile.

unevenly or even wears off entirely. When this happens, bone begins to rub against bone, causing it to get rough or chip away. In some cases, this constant grinding leads to the bony equivalent of scar tissue. The bones grow additional bits of bone, called bone spurs, which can lead to back pain.

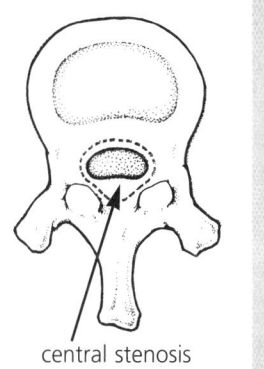

central stenosis

A potentially serious problem that can sometimes result from degenerative changes is called spinal stenosis. This occurs when bone spurs begin growing in such a way that they press against sensitive nerves. When the extra bone grows into the spine and presses against the spinal cord, or cauda equina, it's called central stenosis. When the bone spur grows into smaller nerves where they leave the spinal cord, it's called lateral stenosis. Because spinal stenosis will often put pressure on one or more nerves, it can be very painful, causing shooting pain down one of both legs and even in the hands or arms.

SPINAL STENOSIS

A common reason for shooting leg pain in older adults is pressure on nerves from a back condition called spinal stenosis. Usually caused by a combination of arthritis, bone spurs, and wear and tear on the vertebrae and spinal disks, spinal stenosis results in a narrowing of the spinal canal or other bony passages in the spine.

Other conditions that can cause spinal stenosis include complications from surgery, traumatic injuries, and Paget's disease, in which bone in the spine—as well as in the skull, pelvis, and thighbones—grows beyond its normal boundaries.

SPINAL STENOSIS OR INTERMITTENT CLAUDICATION?

It's not particularly difficult for doctors to identify spinal stenosis. But there's another condition—one that has nothing to do with the spine—that causes similar symptoms.

Intermittent claudication is a disease in which arteries in the legs are partially blocked by fatty deposits. The fat reduces the flow of blood through the arteries, which means that tissues downstream receive less blood and oxygen. Like spinal stenosis, intermittent claudication causes pain in the buttocks, thighs, or calves and makes walking painful.

How can your doctor tell these conditions apart? The best indication, doctors say, is that the pain of intermittent claudication goes away fairly quickly.

One quick test is to head for the grocery store and lean on the guide bar while walking behind your cart. This simple maneuver will often ease the pain of spinal stenosis but won't help with intermittent claudication.

There are two main types of spinal stenosis. One kind, called central stenosis, occurs when bony spurs begin to push their way into the spinal canal. The other, called lateral stenosis, is a bit different. Rather than pressing into the spinal canal itself, the bony growths block smaller channels off to the sides of the canal. When the growths press against nerves inside these channels, pain can shoot to various parts of the body, depending on which nerve has been affected.

Coping with Spinal Stenosis

Since spinal stenosis is usually caused by overgrowths of bone, it's easy to spot with standard medical tests, such as X-ray, computed axial tomography (CAT) scans, magnetic resonance imaging (MRI), or myelogram (a test in which dye is injected into the spinal canal to show whether bony growths are present).

Even without sophisticated tests, your doctor can get a pretty good idea of whether spinal stenosis is causing your pain. One easy test is to have you bend forward. With many back problems, bending forward makes the pain worse. For people with spinal stenosis, however, bending often eases the pain because it widens the spinal canal, relieving pressure on the nerves inside.

When you have spinal stenosis, coughing, sneezing, or even having a bowel movement can be excruciating. And unlike disk problems, which usually cause intermittent pain, the pain of spinal stenosis doesn't go away. As we mentioned earlier, spinal stenosis often causes shooting pain down both legs. (With disk problems, the pain usually affects just one leg.)

When spinal stenosis is severe, your doctor may recommend surgery to trim away the bone that's pressing on the nerves. (For more on decompression surgery, see chapter 5.) Your doctor may also inject an epidural block, a spinal anesthetic that quickly stops the pain, along with steroids to relieve inflammation.

For mild to moderate spinal stenosis, home treatments can be helpful. Lying on your side (but not on your back) will often ease the pain. Back braces are helpful in some cases, as are over-the-counter medications such as aspirin and aspirin substitutes such as acetaminophen or ibuprofen. Your doctor may also recommend stretches and exercises to improve your strength and flexibility, as well as postural training and sometimes a cane to decrease pain and weight bearing on the lower back. And if you're overweight, losing a few pounds will also take some of the strain off your spine, which will help ease the pain.

HERNIATED DISKS

You wouldn't think that something as simple as sneezing or putting away groceries could cause so much pain, but that's often how herniated disks happen. One minute you're feeling just fine, and the next you feel like someone is taking a hammer to your lower back—and pushing knives into your legs or buttocks at the same time.

Separating the spine's 24 vertebrae are spinal disks— the body's equivalent of jelly doughnuts. The outer part of the disk is tough and fibrous. Inside the disk is a softer, gel-like center. (For a complete description of spinal disks, see chapter 1.) The disks act like shock absorbers for the spine. They also help prevent adjoining vertebrae from grinding against each other.

As you get older, the flow of blood nourishing each disk naturally diminishes, causing the soft center to dry out and flatten. The disk gets harder and weaker. What's more, small cracks may appear in the protective outer layer. When that happens, it's like driving a car that has a bulge in the tire—you know you'll be reaching for the jack soon enough.

HOW DISKS HERNIATE

The spinal disks are simply cushions that sit between the vertebrae. They act as shock absorbers and also prevent the vertebrae from rubbing against each other.

Each spinal disk consists of two parts. The outer portion of the disk, called the annulus fibrosus, is made of tough fibers that are interwoven somewhat like the surface of a radial tire. The inner portion of the disk, the nucleus

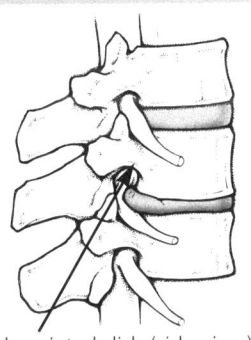

herniated disk (side view)

pulposus, is much softer—more like a gel. The combination of the tough outer layer and the soft middle is what enables the spinal disks to provide so much protection. And because the disks are very flexible, the spine is flexible as well.

When you get older, however, the soft middle of a disk begins to dry out, and the entire disk becomes hard and brittle. Like an old rubber hose, the disk gets fragile and may develop cracks. When this happens, everyday pressure on the spine—from jumping off a step, for example—may cause the disk to herniate. This means that the gel-like material inside pushes its way out. In some cases this merely causes moderate back pain. But if the gel presses against a spinal nerve, the pain can be excruciating. When a disk in the lower back herniates, there may be shooting pain down one or both legs. When a disk in the upper back herniates, there may be pain in the hands or arms.

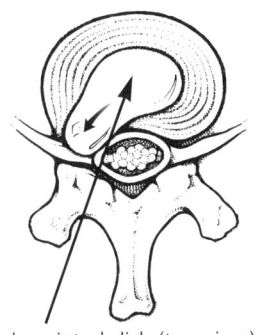

herniated disk (top view)

Even though sneezing (or anything that similarly puts pressure on the spine) doesn't exactly cause disk problems, it can make an already weakened disk rupture, or herniate. When this happens, the gel inside the disk bulges out. If there happens to be a nerve nearby, the gel presses against the nerve, in many instances causing agonizing pain.

Any of the spine's disks can herniate, but the ones most at risk are in the lumbar region of the lower back, where stresses are highest.

Even though herniations occur suddenly, there's usually some warning. In fact, many people will have had several years of intermittent, fairly mild back pain before the disk finally "blows."

Sciatica

One of the most common symptoms of a herniated disk is a condition called sciatica. Sciatica often occurs when one of two spinal nerves gets irritated or inflamed due to pressure from the ruptured disk.

The pain of sciatica can strike different parts of the body, depending on where the nerve is being irritated. A ruptured disk in the lumbar (lower back) region of the spine usually causes pain or numbness in one of your legs or buttocks. If the ruptured disk is in your neck (a cervical disk), you may feel similar pain in your arm and hand. Most cases of sciatica affect the legs (below the knees), however, since herniated lumbar disks are the most common.

A herniated disk is the most common cause of sciatica, but it's not the only one. In older people particularly, sciatica may be caused by spinal stenosis, in which bony spurs press against the nerves.

Sciatica can be terribly painful, but most of the time, the pain doesn't last forever (although it may feel like forever to you). When it's caused by a herniated disk, sciatica

THE CAUSES OF SCIATICA

Nerves are very sensitive, and the slightest pressure can cause excruciating pain. When you're having sciatica, your doctor will want to know what, exactly, is causing the problem. The most common conditions include:

+ A herniated disk
+ Spinal stenosis
+ Vertebral osteomyelitis (a spinal infection)
+ Spondylolisthesis (a type of arthritis)
+ A fractured vertebra
+ A tumor (rarely)

usually lasts about six weeks and then goes away on its own. When it's caused by spinal stenosis, you'll get quicker relief—usually in about a month. In about 25 percent of cases, however, sciatica caused by spinal stenosis will hang on for four months or longer.

If you suspect you have sciatica, you need to see a doctor right away. But you can also test for it yourself. Sciatic pain usually gets better when you straighten your spine—by standing rather than sitting, for example. It tends to get worse when you bend over, raise your leg, or are coughing, sneezing, or having a bowel movement.

Coping with Sciatica and Herniated Disks

Doctors sometimes use sophisticated tests such as MRI to confirm that a disk has ruptured, particularly in cases where diagnosis is difficult. (These tests are also used to pinpoint the problem area prior to surgery.) Doctors see a lot of people with herniated disks, however, and they can often diagnose the problem just by asking some questions and doing a few simple tests.

The pain itself can be a giveaway. People with sciatica, especially younger people, almost always have herniated disks. Another test is to have you lie on your back and raise your leg. When you have sciatica, raising your leg will be very painful.

In addition, nerve problems can cause your reflexes to weaken. Your doctor will check your reflexes on both legs at your knees and ankles, to see if one side is weaker than the other. He might also poke your feet with pins to test for numbness and to test your muscles for strength.

Even though herniated disks are potentially serious, 8 in 10 people who have them won't require surgery. Given time—and a little help from rest, postural exercises, and over-the-counter medications—the pain and inflammation will gradually get better, and the pain will probably go away.

When the pain won't retreat, however, your doctor may inject steroids into the area to bring down the inflammation. And it's possible that you will be among the 20 percent of people with ruptured disks who require surgery. (For a description of the different types of disk surgery, see chapter 5.)

VERTEBRAL COMPRESSION FRACTURES

You can think of your spine as a building with 24 floors—one for each vertebra. Each floor helps support the one above it. But when one floor cracks or collapses, the entire structure is weakened.

Compression fractures are like that. As with any bone, the vertebrae are normally quite strong. But sometimes they are damaged (in an accident, for example), or develop hairline cracks, or even collapse entirely. Whatever the cause, such damage makes the whole spine weaker and causes intense pain and swelling.

Here's a look at the two primary causes of compression fractures: injuries and osteoporosis.

Injuries

In people age 60 and younger, compression fractures are usually caused by accidents—a car crash, for example, or a fall down a flight of stairs. They can also occur during rough-and-tumble sports such as wrestling. Young men have a higher risk of these types of injuries than young women do, probably because they're often likely to be more physically active.

Osteoporosis and Other Causes

As people age, compression fractures are more often caused by bone problems than by accidents. A condition called Paget's disease, for example, causes bones to become thick and almost crumbly, so they're more likely to fracture. Certain steroids used to treat other diseases can cause the bones to weaken. Fractures may also be caused by cancer or by a hormonal problem called hyperparathyroidism, in which a tumor on the parathyroid gland causes it to churn out too much hormone. This in turn reduces the amount of calcium in the bones, making them weaker. Fortunately, each of these conditions is quite rare.

Much more common is osteoporosis, a bone-thinning disease that is the most common cause of fragile bones in older adults, affecting about 28 million people in the United States. Women are especially hard hit. In fact, it is estimated that 50 percent of American women (and 13 percent of men) will have fractures due to osteoporosis during their lifetimes. Coming up, we'll take a closer look at osteoporosis.

As with herniated disks and many other back problems, compression fractures often appear to come out of the blue. Once a vertebra is weakened, it doesn't need much to crack.

A vigorous golf swing or a simple misstep could do the job. The pain usually begins immediately, although some people may not feel it for a few days.

Coping with Vertebral Compression Fractures

Unlike herniated disks, which involve soft tissue, compression fractures involve bone. As a result, they're easy to spot with conventional X-rays.

When compression fractures and the accompanying symptoms are severe—and, in the case of osteoporosis, when they persist despite medical care—your doctor may recommend that you have a spinal fusion. This is a surgical procedure that bonds adjoining vertebrae together to increase strength and stability. Most of the time, however, the pain can be relieved at home.

Taking it easy for a few days will relieve pressure and allow the swelling to go down. Your doctor may give you prescription pain pills, as well.

Once the worst of the pain is gone, all you really need is time to recover. Ice and heat treatments will relieve pain and swelling, and wearing a brace will help keep the spinal column stable.

Although short-term strategies will relieve the pain, you're going to need a long-term plan to resolve the underlying problem—which is weakened bone. Regular exercise, calcium supplements, and in some cases, hormone replacement therapy, are ways to keep osteoporosis under control.

OSTEOPOROSIS

Although there is growing awareness of osteoporosis, many women don't realize they have it until they break a bone for the first time. This is unfortunate because osteoporosis, which causes bones to get weak and soft, can easily be prevented with regular exercise before, during, and after

HOW OSTEOPOROSIS
WEAKENS THE BONES

We think of bones as being nearly indestructible. But, in fact, they're constantly breaking down and building up, a process called remodeling. Remodeling is not only natural but also necessary for survival.

The body uses large amounts of calcium to go about its daily business. It has to get the mineral from somewhere, and bone is the body's calcium bank. Bone is constantly being broken down by specialized cells called osteoclasts. This breaking down is what provides the body with calcium. At the same time, of course, the body is also replacing the bone that's taken away, so the whole process is in equilibrium.

As a woman nears menopause, however, her estrogen levels begin to decline, which causes bones to absorb less calcium. Over time, they begin to weaken and soften, a condition called osteoporosis. When osteoporosis affects the vertebrae, they may get so weak that they begin to develop cracks or even break entirely, causing compression fractures. This is especially common in vertebrae in the chest part of the spine (the thoracic vertebrae).

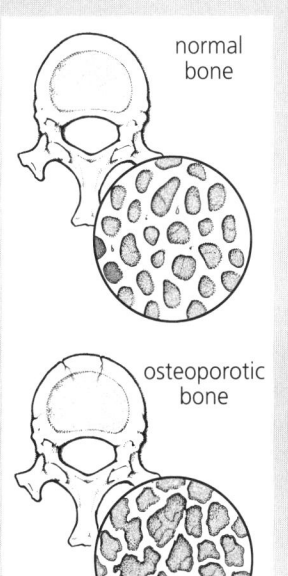

normal bone

osteoporotic bone

Osteoporosis sounds serious— and it is. But it's often easy to prevent simply by getting more calcium in your diet, taking supplements, and exercising. If you do develop osteoporosis, your doctor may also recommend one of the new bone-building drugs such as alendronate (Fosamax).

menopause, along with calcium supplements and hormone replacement therapy. We'll discuss these strategies shortly. But first, let's take a closer look at this bone-breaking condition.

Osteoporosis is primarily a woman's disease. It usually begins after menopause, when a woman's estrogen and calcium levels decline. Doctors aren't sure why, but Caucasian and Asian women have an especially high risk of osteoporosis. In fact, up to 20 million American women either have osteoporosis or are at risk for getting it. The problem has increased dramatically in recent years, partly because we are becoming an older society as the population of elderly people increases. Another reason is that the seats of our pants are usually rooted to the seats of our chairs—we are, unfortunately, more sedentary than ever.

Osteoporosis is one of the leading causes of vertebral compression fractures—and it explains why older women often get shorter with age. When fractures occur in vertebrae in the chest area, women may develop stooped posture from a spinal deformity known as dowager's hump, or kyphosis. Perhaps the most devastating consequence of osteoporosis is hip fractures, which require hospitalization, surgery, and long recuperation and rehabilitation. And at the worst, some fractures can cause nerve or spinal cord pressure that may result in some degree of paralysis.

Apart from these problems, compression fractures may also cause a protuberant abdomen (with a sensation of fullness that can then cause unintended weight loss), weakened spinal muscles, reduced lung capacity, and spinal stenosis.

Coping with Osteoporosis

There's not a lot you can do when bone damage from osteoporosis has already occurred. But there are many ways you can help prevent osteoporosis from getting started.

RISK FACTORS FOR OSTEOPOROSIS

Being a woman automatically puts you at higher risk for developing osteoporosis. Other risk factors include:

- Small frame
- Menopause
- Early onset of menopause (either surgically or naturally)
- Heredity or being of Caucasian or Asian descent
- Low-calcium diet or vitamin D deficiency
- Sedentary lifestyle
- Use of medications such as corticosteroids or anticonvulsants
- Smoking
- Excessive use of alcohol
- Overactive thyroid gland (hyperthyroidism) or excessive thyroid hormone taken for an underactive thyroid
- Rheumatoid arthritis
- Kidney disease
- Testosterone deficiency in men

Boost Your Calcium Intake

The most powerful strategy for preventing and even reversing osteoporosis is to get more calcium—a mineral that is essential for strong bones—in your diet. It's important to start when you're young, since bones begin losing calcium (and strength) by the time a woman reaches age 35.

Doctors recommend that all women get a minimum of 1,200 milligrams of calcium a day, as well as 400 international units of vitamin D, which helps the body absorb calcium. Women who have reached menopause need even more of the mineral—about 1,500 milligrams a day. And if you find it hard to take in enough calcium through food, studies have shown that calcium supplements can slow or stop bone loss and reduce bone fractures even when started up to five years after menopause. (For details on how to boost your calcium stores, along with your vitamin D intake, see chapter 6.)

Exercise Your Bones

For years, doctors were nervous about recommending weight lifting or other forms of weight-bearing exercise for women with osteoporosis because they worried that high stresses could damage bones. Research has shown, however, that the opposite is true. Walking, lifting weights, and riding a bicycle can actually strengthen bones. What's more, women with osteoporosis often feel better and have less back pain when they exercise regularly. And premenopausal women who exercise for 20 minutes a day, at least four times a week, for the 10 years leading up to menopause don't get osteoporosis at all.

Consider Hormone Replacement Therapy

There has been a lot of controversy about hormone replacement therapy (HRT), in which menopausal women are given synthetic forms of estrogen and progesterone to replenish the body's flagging supplies. In terms of back pain, the great advantage of HRT is that it protects you against osteoporosis, reducing your risk of vertebral fractures by as much as 75 percent. Although the sooner you begin HRT after menopause, the more bone you'll preserve, recent studies suggest that HRT can lessen bone loss even when started some years after menopause. Its most powerful benefit, however, may be the protection it gives against heart disease, the number-one killer of women. In addition, HRT can reduce some of the uncomfortable symptoms that occur when menopause begins, such as night sweats and hot flashes.

There has been some concern about evidence of a link between long-term HRT and an increased risk of cancer. These studies are controversial, however. Although estrogen alone does increase the risk of uterine cancer, keeping the dose low and adding a progestin eliminates the added risk. Another factor that complicates the decision, however, is that the risk of breast cancer may increase after 10 to 15 years of HRT.

It's important to discuss the pros and cons of HRT with your doctor. Your own medical history and family history can help guide your decision, as can a bone density test. If osteoporosis and heart disease run in your family, HRT may be a good choice. If you have a family history of breast cancer, your doctor can help you evaluate the risks. She may recommend that you pursue other alternatives.

The bottom line? Although HRT can be a complicated decision (for example, if both heart disease and breast cancer appear on your family tree), most doctors say it is often recommended because heart disease kills many more women than breast cancer does. In other words, you're likely to have a much greater risk of dying from heart disease without HRT than of dying from breast cancer with HRT.

Ask About Bone-Builders

Even if your bones are already showing signs of osteoporosis, your doctor may have some encouraging news for you. New medications for treating osteoporosis have recently been approved by the federal Food and Drug Administration. What's different about these drugs, including alendronate (Fosamax) and calcitonin (Calcimar), is that they can actually build bone.

For an overview of both HRT and these new drugs, see "Drugs to Treat Osteoporosis" on pages 50-51 and also in chapter 9.

DRUGS TO TREAT

Drug Type	Average Daily Dose*	How It Works
Hormone replacement therapy, or HRT (Premarin, Prempro, Provera)	Premarin: 0.625 mg Prempro: made up of 0.625 mg Premarin and 2.5 mg Provera Provera: 2.5 mg or 5 mg	In women, declining estrogen levels after menopause dramatically increase the risk of osteoporosis and fractures. HRT replaces the estrogen no longer produced by the ovaries.
Alendronate (Fosamax)	10 mg	Alendronate—the most potent of the bisphosphonate drugs—inhibits cells that break down bone tissue (osteoclasts) and helps preserve bone mass.
Calcitonin (Calcimar, Miacalcin)	Calcimar: 50 to 100 IU (injected daily or every other day) Miacalcin: 200 IU (1 spray)	Calcitonin—a synthetic protein similar to a hormone produced by the human thyroid gland—inhibits bone resorption and preserves bone mass.

* These dosages represent average ranges for the prevention or treatment of osteoporosis. The precise dosage varies from patient to patient and depends on many factors. Do not make any changes in your medication without consulting your doctor.

OSTEOPOROSIS

Comments	Estimated cost**
Considered the first choice for prevention and treatment of osteoporosis in women. Studies have shown that HRT helps prevent osteoporotic fractures and can reduce bone loss even when begun years after menopause. In addition, HRT has other health benefits—most importantly, the reduction of coronary heart disease risk. The danger of uterine cancer is increased in women using estrogen supplements alone, but HRT combines estrogen with a progestin to neutralize this risk. Those with a strong family or personal history of breast cancer may be unable to take HRT, since it may slightly increase the risk of this disease.	Premarin (0.625 mg) $43.85 Prempro (0.625 mg/2.5 mg) $68.58 Provera (2.5 mg) $40.41; (5 mg) $57.03
Studies have shown that alendronate reduces the risk of fractures. A major side effect of alendronate—inflammation of the esophagus, which can lead to heartburn or ulcers—can often be prevented by taking the drug with a full glass of water first thing in the morning (at least 30 minutes before breakfast) and remaining upright (sitting or standing) for at least 30 minutes afterward. Other side effects include gastrointestinal problems, such as abdominal pain, nausea, constipation, and diarrhea, but usually only with very high doses.	Fosamax (10 mg) $172.96
While calcitonin has not been proven to reduce fracture risk, studies have shown that it can increase bone density. It is recommended for those who cannot or will not take HRT as well as for those with low bone mass more than five years after menopause. The drug appears particularly helpful for those with chronic pain from vertebral compression fractures. Side effects include nausea, loss of appetite, flushing, and, with the nasal spray form, nasal irritation or dryness.	Calcimar (400 IU's) $46.58 Miacalcin (200 IU's) $50.06

** *These are wholesale prices to pharmacists for 100 tablets or capsules (or for daily injections, where indicated) of the dosage strengths listed in parentheses. Costs to consumers are higher. Source: Red Book, 1997 (Medical Economics Company).*

ARTHRITIC DISEASES OF THE SPINE

Your body's immune system is a powerful ally. It stops bacteria and viruses before they make you sick, and it even helps battle cancer cells before they have a chance to spread. Sometimes, however, the immune system gets confused. Rather than attacking only invaders, it turns its formidable powers inward and begins attacking you. Conditions that cause this situation are known as autoimmune diseases.

Rheumatoid arthritis, a common autoimmune disease, sometimes damages bones in the spine, causing pain as well as a breakdown of bone and cartilage. Another form of arthritis, called ankylosing spondylitis, acts in similar ways.

Not all forms of arthritis are caused by the immune system, however. One of the most common forms of arthritis, called osteoarthritis, occurs any time there is stress or strain in a joint. In the spine, it is usually related to the changes that come with aging. Osteoarthritis can be quite painful, but it usually is less destructive than the autoimmune forms of arthritis.

Ankylosing Spondylitis

A uniquely painful and serious form of arthritis is a condition called ankylosing spondylitis. It causes the facet joints of the vertebrae—as well as the sacroiliac joints at the hips—to become painfully inflamed. Nearby ligaments and tendons may also get sore and swollen.

This type of arthritis is usually hereditary and tends to affect men in their twenties and thirties. It usually comes on slowly and gets worse over time, causing stiffness and lower back pain, especially in the mornings. In severe cases, damage to the vertebrae can cause them to fuse together, forming a stiff, rod-like back that makes movement difficult. And if ankylosing spondylitis is very serious, it may lead to severe deformities that usually must be corrected with surgery.

Unlike many causes of back pain, ankylosing spondylitis tends to be less painful when you exercise. Bed rest often makes it worse.

Rheumatoid Arthritis

Like ankylosing spondylitis, rheumatoid arthritis causes joint pain and swelling. Rather than affecting the spine, however, it usually damages small joints in the hands and the neck (or cervical spine), elbows, and knees. When rheumatoid arthritis does strike, it can be extremely serious, literally deforming and destroying joints and making movement difficult and very painful.

Osteoarthritis

Known as wear-and-tear arthritis, osteoarthritis occurs in almost all of us as we get older. After years of twisting, turning, and bending, joints in the spine begin to wear, which can make us sore and creaky.

Osteoarthritis in the spine isn't usually serious. Most of the time, in fact, it causes only minor aches and pains. For some people, however, the wear and tear can cause serious damage. When that happens, the spine can become extremely stiff and painful.

Coping with Arthritis

There isn't a real cure for any of these forms of arthritis. While regular exercise can relieve some of the pain and stiffness, it can't repair damage that has already been done.

Over-the-counter and prescription medications provide some relief for ankylosing spondylitis (as well as for osteoarthritis). When the problem is severe, however, surgery to repair the joints—or at least to remove bits of bone that are causing pain—may be the best option.

Rheumatoid arthritis is tricky to treat. Over-the-counter medications to relieve pain and swelling can be very effective, at least at first. If the condition gets worse—as it often does—you may need stronger medications, possibly including drugs that suppress the immune system in order to stop the attacks. Sometimes surgery is recommended to relieve neck pain or pressure on the nerves.

SPONDYLOLISTHESIS

Despite the tongue-twisting name, this condition has a fairly simple cause. Some people will develop a defect in a vertebra (called spondylolysis) that causes the bone to weaken—just as a crockery pot with a hairline crack is weak. If the vertebra is sufficiently damaged, the facet joints can simply break away.

Some people won't have symptoms for years. But eventually, the weak bones can separate, causing the vertebrae to slip forward. (Doctors call this forward subluxation.) The slippage usually occurs at the base of the lumbar (lower back) spine. As the vertebrae slip out of place, the spine's natural alignment is thrown out of balance, straining the ligaments and joints. About 75 percent of people with this condition experience chronic pain. And in some cases, the slipping vertebrae press against the sciatic nerves, causing pain in the legs as well.

Some children are born with spondylolysis and may have no symptoms throughout their lives. In adults, it may be caused by injuries, normal wear and tear, or conditions such as arthritis and diabetes. It may also occur in divers, gymnasts, and other athletes who stretch out their backs well beyond the normal range. Competitive weight lifters are also at risk because of the enormous strain they put on their backs.

Coping with Spondylolisthesis

This condition can readily be diagnosed with X-rays. The treatments, however, aren't so simple. Wearing a back brace and taking medications help some people, but not everyone.

Surgery, however, can often be effective. The most common operation is called spinal fusion, in which vertebrae are fused together, making the spine more stable. In some cases, simply removing part of a vertebra that's pressing against a nerve relieves the pain. (For more information on spinal fusion, see chapter 5.)

SPINAL DEFORMITIES

It would be nice if the spine always maintained a perfect S-shaped curve. But sometimes it will bend or twist at odd angles, causing a painful strain on the back.

There are several types of spinal deformities. Here are the most common.

Kyphosis

Often referred to as dowager's hump or humpback, this condition exaggerates the curve of the spine in the upper back, giving it a humplike appearance. Kyphosis may occur when a number of vertebrae collapse—usually because of osteoporosis. It can also develop in tall people, some of whom try to appear shorter by stooping and rolling their shoulders forward. Sometimes it can result from birth defects or growth problems in young adolescents.

Not surprisingly, the stooped-over position of kyphosis can result in back pain. More seriously, it can also shorten some of the chest muscles, making the chest cavity smaller. This in turn can make breathing difficult because the lungs have less room in which to expand.

Kyphosis can sometimes be reversed through exercise and lessons in proper posture. More severe cases, however, generally require surgery to straighten the spine.

Lordosis

This is a less common condition in which the spine assumes a swaybacked shape. Sometimes caused by a lifetime of poor posture, overweight, or structural misalignments of the spine, lordosis throws the entire spine off balance, putting pressure on the spinal disks and also on the facet joints. People with lordosis often have lower back pain and sometimes sciatica as well. Improving your posture will often help reverse this condition.

Scoliosis

Most common in teenaged girls, scoliosis is a condition in which the back is curved or twisted to the side, often giving a stooped appearance. Some people are born with scoliosis. But more often, and for unknown reasons, it begins around puberty—at the same time as or just before a girl's secondary sexual characteristics, such as breast development, begin to appear. If it's not corrected at an early age, scoliosis can cause some muscles to tighten and shorten, while other muscles stretch and grow weak. Because scoliosis changes the shape of the chest cavity, the lungs and heart may be affected.

When scoliosis is caught early, it's usually easy to stop its progress by wearing a brace, if needed. In addition, doctors usually recommend exercises to help stretch and strengthen the affected muscles.

It's also possible for scoliosis to appear for the first time later in life, after age 50. These cases are usually the result of asymmetric, or unevenly balanced, wear on the body's joints, which can bend the spine over time.

Coping with Spinal Deformities

The one good thing about spinal deformities is that pain isn't always a problem. When it is, over-the-counter anti-inflammatory medications can usually take care of it. Surgery is needed only when the condition is unusually severe, seems to be getting worse, or is causing pain.

FIBROMYALGIA

Unlike many back problems, fibromyalgia isn't caused by damage to bones or joints. Fibromyalgia is a collection of symptoms that, taken together, are considered a syndrome, not a disease. Found in women more often than men, it usually occurs between the ages of 20 and 50, and may affect as many as two percent of Americans. Fibromyalgia triggers pain in muscles, tendons, and ligaments, rather than in the joints, and also causes fatigue. Often it will trigger depression as well, particularly because of the frustrating symptoms, but also because the condition is poorly understood and difficult to diagnose. Some researchers think it's caused by small traumas to the muscles—which may occur after flu, or extreme physical or emotional stress—that decrease the blood flow. Others believe that the root of the disease is a sleep disorder that often occurs simultaneously. For some reason, in people with fibromyalgia, the deepest and most restful cycle of sleep is interrupted, although they might not be aware of it. Significantly, even healthy people showed symptoms of fibromyalgia when they were deprived of this type of sleep.

Coping with Fibromyalgia

Fibromyalgia is usually diagnosed by pressing on 18 of the body's tender points. If pressing on these predetermined points causes pain, your doctor will likely suspect that you have this condition.

The best treatment for fibromyalgia is exercise, doctors say. Gentle aerobic activity, such as treadmill walking, biking, or swimming, is the basic strategy. In some cases, tender points are injected with medication or pressure is applied to relieve pain. Afterwards, a consistent stretching program is essential. If sleep is difficult, tricyclic antidepressants (in lower doses than are prescribed for depression) have been proven to help restore normal sleep patterns.

If you have fibromyalgia and your doctor feels that stress, depression, or anxiety may be aggravating your pain, she may also recommend relaxation training or another appropriate therapy. And, although many alternative therapists tout the results of their home remedies for fibromyalgia syndrome, be sure to discuss any such treatment with your doctor. None has been formally studied for safety or effectiveness, and some may be harmful.

OSTEOMALACIA

This condition is most likely to occur in adults. It is similar to rickets, a condition in children that is caused by poor nutrition.

Osteomalacia—which can cause bone fractures as well as back, rib, and pelvic pain—is the softening of bone that occurs when there's a shortage of calcium and phosphorus in the body. Vitamin D deficiency is a major cause of osteomalacia because vitamin D supports calcium absorbtion. Other causes are chronically low levels of phosphate in the body, poor absorption of calcium, and decreased mineralization. Mineralization is the building process that takes place when the two components of bone—minerals and fibers called collagen—come together. The minerals affix to the collagen fibers, hardening the bone.

Osteomalacia isn't always caused by a poor diet, however. Liver disease, alcohol abuse, certain antacid medications, and insufficient exposure to sunlight can also cause vitamin D levels to drop.

Coping with Osteomalacia

Osteomalacia isn't very common. But once its cause is discovered, it can be treated by increasing the amount of vitamin D and calcium in the diet, by taking prescribed vitamin and mineral supplements, and by eliminating alcohol.

VERTEBRAL OSTEOMYELITIS

A bacterial infection of the spine, vertebral osteomyelitis is not only painful but, in some cases, very difficult to treat. It often causes a fever as well as pain in the back or neck.

Vertebral osteomyelitis sometimes occurs after spinal surgery, when bacteria get inside the spinal canal. More often it's caused by an infection elsewhere in the body (such as in the kidneys or bladder) that travels to the spine. People with diabetes or other diseases that lower immune resistance are at higher risk for osteomyelitis. The problem is rapidly increasing, doctors say, as the population ages and immune deficiencies become more common.

Coping with Vertebral Osteomyelitis

Prompt treatment of osteomyelitis is crucial because the condition can damage the vertebrae and also cause abscesses within the spine.

Doctors can diagnose osteomyelitis with MRI as well as by taking a biopsy from the affected area. When the infection is caught early, antibiotics will clear it up. In some cases, however, surgery is required to remove damaged bone and other tissue and to clean out the infected area.

Cauda Equina Syndrome

At the base of the spinal cord is a thick bundle of nerves that looks just like a horse's tail—which is what the term *cauda equina* means. Problems occur when something—a ruptured spinal disk, for example—presses against the bundle of nerves.

Cauda equina syndrome, while rare, is always an emergency. It can cause a loss of bowel or bladder control, numbness in the groin, buttocks, and legs, and weakness or paralysis of the leg muscles. It's vital to seek treatment immediately if you experience any of these symptoms.

Coping with Cauda Equina Syndrome

Surgery to remove whatever is causing the pressure is the only treatment for cauda equina syndrome. Once the underlying problem has been taken care of, the pain should clear up very quickly.

Cancer

Fortunately, cancer of the back is quite rare. When it does occur, it usually causes pain around the mid-back. It can cause sciatic nerve pain as well. People with cancer of the back usually have worse pain when they're active, but the pain isn't relieved by lying down.

Cancer of the back is usually caused by metastasis—that is, when a tumor elsewhere in the body sends cancer cells to the back. Breast and prostate cancers are the most common causes of such metastases. An exception is a type of cancer called multiple myeloma, in which cancer cells from bone marrow travel to the spine and form a tumor there.

The frightening thing about myeloma is that the symptoms often are very similar to those caused by other, less serious conditions, such as vertebral compression fractures. That's why it's always important to see your doctor when back pain doesn't get better within 7 to 10 days.

Coping with Cancer

Obviously, cancer isn't a condition you can treat on your own. Depending on the type of cancer and where it's found, your doctor may recommend chemotherapy, radiation, or surgery.

OTHER SYSTEMIC DISEASES

Most back pain, naturally enough, begins in the back. But sometimes problems in other parts of your body can cause what doctors call referred back pain. People with kidney infections, for example, may develop pain in the small of the back. The same is true of gallstones, ulcers, and many other conditions. Once the underlying problem is taken care of, the back pain will quickly go away.

HEALING WITH TIME

As we've seen, there are many causes of back pain. Some are minor and easy to fix; others are much more challenging. What they have in common is a sneaky streak: Even for doctors who specialize in back problems, each new case can leave them baffled.

But don't forget that serious back problems are the easiest to diagnose—which means you'll get the best care very quickly. As for back pains that aren't so serious, they'll generally go away on their own within a few days or weeks. What this means, of course, is that it won't take long to put your back pain behind you!

CHAPTER THREE

Finding Medical Care

We usually treat back pain a lot like a winter cold: Spend some time in bed, take a day or two off from work, and generally lie low until it runs its course.

That's not a bad approach, because 4 in 10 back problems go away within a week, and 9 in 10 get better within two months. Of course, it can feel like a long two months. Back pain hurts—sometimes just a little, but usually a lot. In most cases, however, a combination of time, mild anti-inflammatory drugs, and a few days spent watching daytime TV will take out the kinks.

But sometimes the pain doesn't get better or, more frightening, gets even worse. What began as a minor backache can turn into something else—shooting pain down the legs, for example, or even a loss of bladder control. And sometimes the pain just keeps coming back. That's when it's time to put away the ice packs and call your doctor.

Doctors have a lot of experience treating back pain. After asking some questions, rapping a few tendons to check your reflexes, and ordering a test or two, your doctor will have a pretty good idea of what's going on. Even though back pain is notoriously difficult to diagnose with certainty, it's not usually that hard to design a treatment plan to ease the pain—and, just as importantly, to prevent additional problems from coming at you down the road.

In the following pages, we'll take a look behind the scenes. We'll discuss the most common tests doctors use (and when they're right for you), the best specialists for your condition, and when you may want to consider getting complementary medical care. Back pain can be exceedingly complex. This chapter will make it a little bit clearer.

WHEN TO SEE YOUR DOCTOR

Sometimes you may find it hard to judge whether your back needs professional attention or whether simple home remedies—resting a little, taking over-the-counter pain pills, and applying cold packs or hot pads—will do the trick. Most backaches respond well to these sorts of treatments. Others, unfortunately, do not.

When back pain is severe and lasts for more than 7 to 10 days, it's time to pick up the phone and call your doctor. You shouldn't wait even that long if you've been in an accident or if there are other symptoms besides pain. (See "Serious Warning Signs.") Back pain is often accompanied by injuries to the nerves, and fast treatment may be essential to prevent the problem from getting worse.

THE FIRST STOP: YOUR FAMILY DOCTOR

Most episodes of back pain don't require a visit to a specialist. Your family doctor probably sees as many sore backs as sore throats. In almost all cases, he'll be able to successfully treat the problem.

Doctors get a lot of training in treating back pain, and they have an impressive arsenal of techniques for treating it—everything from prescription drugs to physical therapy, electrical stimulation, and even massage.

In recent years, there has been a surge of interest in alternative treatments for back pain. Chiropractic, acupressure, acupuncture, and other kinds of alternative care can

SERIOUS WARNING SIGNS

Back pain is almost always intense no matter what causes it. You can't always use how much it hurts as a guide to whether or not the problem is serious. However, certain symptoms are always warning signs. Doctors estimate that 2 percent of backaches should be seen by a physician right away. You should call your doctor immediately if you experience any of the following:

- You can't bend from the waist.
- You have a limp.
- The pain is constant and severe and lasts for more than two days.
- The pain doesn't get better when you change positions.
- There's shooting pain, numbness, tingling, or weakness in your hands, back, buttocks, legs, or feet.
- It hurts when you lift your leg straight up.
- You've had a loss of bowel or bladder control.
- The pain continues even when you're getting rest, including at night.
- You've had repeated episodes of severe pain.
- You are losing weight or have a fever.

be helpful for some people. But you should always begin by seeing your regular doctor. Alternative therapies don't work—or, worse, may even be dangerous—for some kinds of back pain. This is especially true when you have a serious condition such as a herniated disk or a vertebral compression fracture. Undergoing back manipulations when you have one of these conditions can make the problem much worse.

Even though your doctor has (or has access to) enough machines, gizmos, and gadgets to fill a science fiction movie, one of the most powerful tools is also the simplest. It's called your medical history, and it's the cornerstone of any back care plan. Your medical history does more than help your doctor understand what may have caused the problem and what the best treatments are. It also provides valuable clues as to whether you'll need specialized tests or a referral to a back pain specialist.

YOUR MEDICAL HISTORY

Even though back pain is easy to recognize, the underlying causes are much more mysterious. To find a solution, your doctor is going to ask you a lot of questions. Where does it hurt? When does it hurt? When did the pain begin? How much does it hurt? Does it hurt when you bend over or when you stand up? The answers to these and dozens of other questions will give your doctor a clearer sense of what the problem actually is.

The medical history doesn't begin and end with the obvious symptom, pain. Your body is much more complex than that. Different types of back pain affect different parts of your body—which is why your doctor will ask about a wide range of symptoms that seemingly have nothing to do with your back.

Symptoms such as numbness or shooting pain in the legs and a loss of bowel or bladder function can tell a lot about what's causing your back pain and how serious it's likely to be. In addition, previous medical problems may play a direct role in some kinds of back pain.

Your lifestyle and personal habits will also be discussed. Someone who lifts boxes for a living, for example, may have a different kind of back pain than someone who sits at a desk. Do you do a lot of bending or twisting? Do you run, swim, or lift weights? Do you smoke? Do you love your job or loathe it? Are you having problems at home? Research has shown that people with a lot of stress in their lives tend to have more problems with back pain than people who don't, so the answers to these questions can be very important.

Finally, your doctor is going to ask you questions that will seem, well, scary. Even though back pain is rarely caused by conditions such as cancer and spinal infections, it's important to find out early on if you're going to need specialized—and possibly emergency—care.

The questions asked during a medical history will vary from person to person—and also from doctor to doctor. Regardless of the questions, the goal of a medical history is to identify your problem and map out a course of treatment. The answers you give will help your doctor decide if you have a complicated condition that requires the attention of a neurologist, an orthopedic surgeon, or another specialist. They'll also help your doctor decide if you need additional tests.

Some questions you'll probably be asked include:

- Where is your pain located? Is it only in the lower back? Does it affect any other area of the back? Does it extend down to the buttocks or legs?
- How severe is your pain? Is it so bad that you can't move? Are you able to do your usual daily activities? Can you drive? Does the pain prevent you from engaging in vigorous activity? More specifically, do you have trouble with only a certain activity, such as golf or gardening?
- Is there anything that makes the pain better or worse? Conditions such as spinal stenosis, for example, are often relieved by bending over and sitting down. A herniated disk, however, often causes more pain when you bend or sit.
- What were you doing when the pain began? Pain that occurs after vigorous activity, for example, is often caused by a sprain or strain. Pain that comes on gradually, however, is usually due to a chronic problem, such a herniated disk or a vertebral compression fracture.

- Is this your first bout with back pain, or has there been a prior episode? If so, how was it treated? How long did it last? How effective was the treatment?
- Do you have any other health problems? There are a number of diseases, including cancer, osteoporosis, and endocrine (hormone) problems, that can damage the spine.
- Are you taking any medications? Some drugs, such as steroids, can cause bones in the spine to weaken.
- What kind of work do you do? How do you spend your leisure time? Back injuries are frequently linked to a particular activity, such as heavy lifting, a sedentary lifestyle, or even spending a lot of time in the car.

As you can see, taking a medical history is an involved process. But it actually goes quite quickly. Within a few minutes, your doctor will know a great deal about you. He won't yet know for sure what the problem is, but he'll have a good idea which direction to go for additional answers.

THE PHYSICAL EXAMINATION

After your doctor has completed the medical history, it's time to get undressed (if you haven't done so already). But don't jump on the table just yet. Your doctor may ask you to stand, bend, or walk around while he looks for problems with your posture, the curvature of your spine, and your overall mobility. An unequal leg length can also predispose you to low back pain. You might have to do some acrobatics as well, such as walking on your tiptoes or heels or bending over sideways.

Now it's time to get on the table (although your doctor may simply sit in a chair while you stand in front of him). Your doctor will feel your back to see if there are tender areas. Tenderness may be a sign of a herniated disk, a compression fracture, a spinal infection or, much more rarely, a tumor.

The location of the tenderness tells a lot about what the problem could be. If you have a herniated disk, for instance, there's a good chance you'll be sensitive near the lumbar (lower back) spine. If you have the condition called ankylosing spondylitis, on the other hand, you may be sore around the sacroiliac joint near the base of your spine. In many cases, of course, tenderness simply means you've strained or sprained your back.

And remember, back pain doesn't always originate in the back. Don't be surprised if your doctor feels around the groin, abdomen, or pelvis, or probes with his fingers to see if there's tenderness in the area of the kidneys or rectum. Tenderness in the abdomen, for example, could be a sign of an abdominal aortic aneurysm—a weak spot in a major artery called the aorta.

Once this general exam is completed, your doctor will perform two of the most important tests for diagnosing back pain: the SLR (straight leg raise) test and the neurological exam.

The SLR Test

It's the simplest test imaginable—and also the most revealing. Your doctor will ask you to lie on your back. He'll lift your legs, one at a time, without bending the knees. The idea is to see if raising your legs causes either pain or a pins-and-needles sensation.

The SLR test is used to reveal the presence of nerve problems. If you have a herniated disk in your lower back, raising your leg will put pressure on a nerve (the sciatic nerve), causing pain or other symptoms. The earlier you experience pain while your leg is being raised, the more serious the disk herniation probably is.

Since the SLR deliberately puts pressure on a possibly inflamed nerve, the test is going to be uncomfortable, and you should be prepared. The upside? It's very accurate. What's more, it provides a benchmark for further testing. Your doctor will probably have you repeat this test as your treatment continues. As time goes by, he should be able to raise your leg higher and higher before the pain starts to kick in.

The Neurological Examination

It's not uncommon for back problems to affect the nerves. The neurological examination will test your strength, reflexes, and sensations in different parts of your body. This will reveal which nerves are being affected by your problem. Neurological tests are especially useful in the diagnosis of herniated disks and spinal stenosis.

A number of nerves branch off from the spine and travel to other areas of the body. These nerves control sensations as well as muscle strength. If a nerve is pinched or compressed as it leaves the spine, the pain can be severe. What's more, the pain doesn't necessarily occur in the exact spot where the nerve is pinched. Instead, the pain signals can travel along the length of the nerve, appearing in the hands, feet, legs, or other parts of your body.

Doctors know a lot about how (and where) nerve pain travels. By identifying where the pain is, your doctor will have a very good idea of where in the spine the problem is originating.

Suppose, for example, you have the condition called sciatica—nerve pain traveling from the spine down one or both legs. If you have pain in only one leg, your doctor will suspect that the sciatica is caused by a herniated disk in your lower back. If you have pain in both legs, the cause of the sciatica is more likely to be spinal stenosis, a narrowing of the spinal canal.

Nerve problems may do more than just cause pain. In some cases, for example, pressure on a nerve causes a loss of bladder control. This usually occurs when a disk has ruptured in the sacral area of the spine, below the lumbar (lower back) region. Similarly, reduced reflexes in your ankles or feet also provide clues as to where the problem is. Even though there isn't a single neurological test that's a perfect measure of back problems, as a group the results can be very helpful.

LABORATORY TESTS

A medical history and physical exam are all it takes to diagnose most back problems (although additional tests may be used to confirm the diagnosis). Unless your symptoms are truly serious, you won't need sophisticated testing. Such tests aren't usually needed and, in some cases, may actually do harm.

Here's why. The back is a complicated piece of equipment, and there's a lot that doctors don't understand. Some people have terrible pain, yet medical tests show that everything is normal. Conversely, some people have actual back damage but suffer no symptoms whatsoever.

For example, doctors have found that when people undergo the test called magnetic resonance imaging (MRI), a good number of them show minor bulges or herniations in the spinal disks. This is true even in people who don't have back pain. So even though herniated disks are a common cause of back pain—as well as of expensive medical treatment—they can also be a normal part of aging.

Suppose you do have back pain and the tests also show you have a herniated disk. There's probably a connection, right? Not necessarily. It's possible that the disk and your pain are entirely unrelated. But tests are hard to ignore, and this type of "false-positive" reading can lead to unnecessary (and costly) procedures when none is actually needed.

Doctors are well aware of these limitations, of course, and they do their best to order additional tests only when they're really useful. And make no mistake: Some back problems are so serious that it's essential to get an accurate diagnosis as soon as possible, no matter how many tests that takes.

Severe nerve pain is a good example. Even though it may clear up on its own, sometimes it doesn't—or it gets progressively worse. Unless the cause of the pain is taken care of, the nerve could be seriously injured, causing permanent damage. For conditions such as this, your doctor will almost certainly want to do additional tests. The same is true if your doctor suspects that a systemic disease such as cancer or infection is the source of your back pain.

People who may need surgery are the ones most likely to be given sophisticated tests such as computed axial tomography (CAT) scans or MRI. For one thing, their doctors will want to know how serious the problem is and whether or not they need to move quickly. In addition, these and other tests can help surgeons "see" the problem area beforehand, so they'll know exactly what they need to do (and where they'll need to go) during surgery.

Doctors today have access to an impressive battery of sophisticated tests, and the technology is getting better all the time. Tests that are commonly used for back problems include imaging studies (such as X-rays, CAT scans, MRI, and myelograms), bone scans, electrical tests, blood and urine tests, and bone density tests.

Imaging Studies

For decades X-rays have been one of the backbones of medicine. Along with more modern imaging studies, such as MRI and CAT scans, X-rays look inside your body, providing an actual picture of the underlying problem.

Imaging studies are essential for diagnosing many back problems. They help your doctor understand the extent of the problem and whether or not further treatment is needed.

In addition, surgeons depend on imaging studies to tell them where to cut and what they're likely to find inside.

Different imaging studies have different strengths and weaknesses. X-rays, for example, are excellent at revealing bone problems but less effective for soft tissue injuries. MRI, by contrast, excels at revealing problems in muscles, ligaments, and other soft tissues.

Here's a look at the most common imaging studies, along with explanations of which back problems they're most likely to be used for.

X-rays

X-rays have been in daily use for decades, and they're still considered one of the best (and also one of the least expensive) ways to reveal a variety of bone disorders. X-rays excel in detecting vertebral compression fractures as well as myeloma, a cancer that invades the bony parts of the spine. They can also reveal spinal stenosis, although other imaging studies do a better job of that.

What X-rays won't do is detect problems in muscles, ligaments, and other soft tissues.

One problem with X-rays is that they tend to be overused. Studies have shown that chiropractors, for example, are apt to order X-rays for routine cases of back pain. Since 90 percent of back pain cases will go away on their own, taking X-rays in the early stages is often a waste of time and money.

There's also the safety issue. Even though modern X-rays are very safe, there's simply no reason to unnecessarily expose yourself to radiation. Finally, X-rays, as with other imaging studies, occasionally will reveal common spinal abnormalities that could be a problem but probably aren't. This can be misleading and may at times lead to unnecessary treatment.

Nonetheless, X-rays are a relatively simple and effective way to verify problems such as fractures. X-rays are widely available and, at $150 to $200 each, are the least expensive of all the imaging studies.

THE BEST USES FOR X-RAYS

X-rays are a powerful diagnostic tool. They're usually used to diagnose these conditions.

- Injuries from traumas—car accidents, for example—that are causing acute pain
- Multiple myeloma and other tumors of the spine
- Vertebral compression fractures
- Ankylosing spondylitis
- Osteomyelitis

CAT Scans

More sensitive than X-rays, CAT scans are often used to detect herniated disks and spinal stenosis. Since they're more expensive than X-rays, they tend to be used for long-standing problems or when X-rays haven't been effective or aren't considered appropriate.

Like X-rays, CAT scans beam radiation through the body in order to detect bone problems. They can also detect some soft tissue injuries. CAT scans provide tremendous detail, and surgeons often depend on them to learn what they're going to encounter in the operating room. CAT scans excel at revealing changes in the vertebrae that may be caused by tumors or infections.

When you get a CAT scan, you lie flat on a table while X-rays are passed through your body and picked up by a sensor rotating around you. The images are then shipped to a computer, which creates a variety of "viewpoints"—

cross-sectional as well as two- and three-dimensional. CAT scans cost approximately $550.

MRI

The safest and most sensitive imaging technique available today is the MRI. More sensitive than CAT scans and X-rays, MRI is able to detect soft tissue problems as well as problems affecting the bones. It is commonly used to diagnose herniated disks and spinal stenosis. It can also pick up signs of osteomyelitis (a spinal infection), tumors, compression of the spinal cord, and abscesses.

Unlike X-rays and CAT scans, MRI doesn't use radiation. Instead, it surrounds your body with a powerful magnetic field while radio waves pass through your body. MRI is painless, but can be uncomfortable because the test takes place inside a hollow tube and lasts for 30 to 60 minutes. For people who are claustrophobic, the test can be extremely unsettling.

Doctors often recommend that people who are claustrophobic try meditation or visualization—a technique in which you fill your mind with soothing images—while the MRI is going on. You can also ask your doctor for a mild tranquilizer.

As with other imaging techniques, MRI tends to be used more than is really necessary. And because it's so sensitive it may detect even slight changes in the body—changes that may not be a problem even though they're not "normal." Studies have shown, for example, that MRI shows herniated disks in as many as 30 percent of people who don't have back pain. This number is even higher when the tests involve older people, who naturally have more degenerative changes.

As you would expect, MRI is expensive, costing between $800 and $1,000. It cannot be used if you have a pacemaker, a metal implant in your body close to the area being studied, or an intrauterine device (IUD).

Myelogram

Most imaging tests are noninvasive—that is, they take pictures of the body without actually breaking the skin or going inside. The myelogram is different. In this test, a dye or contrast material is injected into the spinal canal. The liquid flows into the canal, providing a clear picture of the soft tissues as well as the surrounding bones. Today, myelograms are usually done in combination with a CAT scan for best results.

Myelograms are usually used to diagnose spinal cord problems, although they may be used for herniated disks as well. They're not given routinely, however, but mainly when serious nerve damage is suspected. People who have weakness in the legs or a loss of bowel or bladder control are often given myelograms.

Even though myelograms are extremely effective, they're rarely a doctor's first choice. Although the test itself is painless, the contrast material that's injected into the spinal canal can cause nausea and headaches as well as backaches. As with any invasive procedure, there's a very, very slight risk of infection. Finally, the test is somewhat complicated. People having myelograms must sit or lie with their heads elevated for six to eight hours after the contrast material is injected. The test itself costs about $600.

Bone Scans

If your doctor suspects you have a bone problem—a fractured vertebra, for example, or excessive growth of bone into the spinal canal—he may recommend a bone scan. (Despite the name, bone scans are also used to detect tumors and infections in the spine.)

A bone scan measures bone turnover—the rate at which bone is lost and replaced in your body. The test requires an injection of a radioactive substance called technetium. Two or three hours after the injection, the radioactivity of the spinal bones is measured with a gamma counter, which reveals how fast bone is coming and going.

Bone scans are somewhat uncomfortable. They take three to four hours to complete, and you need to lie on your stomach for about an hour of this time. They usually cost about $300, and the test may not be covered by insurance.

Electrical Tests

The messages that travel to and from your brain—everything from pain signals to instructions to lift your leg—are transmitted through nerves. Certain back problems, such as a ruptured disk or spinal stenosis, often put pressure on spinal nerves, causing pain and slowing the rate at which messages travel.

Electrical tests—these include electromyography, nerve conduction, and sensory-evoked potentials—are most often used when you've been having leg pain, numbness, or weakness for more than a month. The tests allow your doctor to tell if the symptoms are caused by problems in the back or by something that's originating elsewhere in the body, such as diabetes.

The tests usually cost about $750. There is some debate about how useful these tests are. They're usually used only when other tests haven't given conclusive results or when a thorough physical exam is impossible, due to pain, for example.

Blood Tests

Blood tests aren't generally used for the diagnosis of back problems. But they can be helpful in pinpointing a few more serious problems, which are, fortunately, quite rare.

- A blood count—counting the various cells in a blood sample—can reveal a spinal infection such as osteomyelitis.
- A blood test called the erythrocyte sedimentation rate is used to diagnose inflammation, such as that caused by ankylosing spondylitis.
- High levels of a blood component called serum globulin can indicate the presence of myeloma, a bone cancer.
- High levels of an enzyme called alkaline phosphatase are a sign of Paget's disease and other diseases, which can cause excessive bone growth into the spinal canal.
- High levels of calcium are a sign of a hormonal problem called hyperparathyroidism, which causes calcium to be removed from bones, making them weak and brittle.
- High levels of immune system cells called prostate-specific antigens can indicate prostate cancer, which sometimes causes back pain.
- High levels of uric acid are a sign of gout, a type of arthritis that may cause back pain.

Urine Tests

As with blood tests, urine tests aren't commonly used for back pain. But they may be helpful. For example, the presence of abnormal proteins in the urine may be a sign of myeloma, a type of bone cancer. In addition, doctors may look for increased levels of two other substances called hydroxyproline and pyridinoline, that are excreted in the urine. Created by the formation and resorption of bone, these substances are signs of the disease activity seen in osteoporosis and Paget's disease.

Bone Density Tests

Bones are surprisingly strong. At least, they're supposed to be. But in some people—especially women with osteoporosis—the bones become thin and weak and likely to break. Osteoporosis is the main cause of vertebral compression fractures, in which vertebrae crack and even crumble, weakening the spine.

Bone density tests, which measure the strength and density of the bones, make it possible to know what state your bones are in before you actually break one. While X-rays can detect large amounts of bone loss, they're much less sensitive than bone density tests.

A common bone density test is called dual energy X-ray absorptiometry. This test aims two X-rays at the spine or other bones. A computer measures the amount of energy that passes through the bones. When bones are strong and

---

TESTING OPTIONS

Doctors have developed a number of tests for measuring bone density in the spine. The test that's normally used is dual energy X-ray absorptiometry, or DEXA. Others include:

- Dual photon absorptiometry
- Quantitative computed tomography (QCT)
- Peripheral QCT
- Radiographic absorptiometry
- Single energy X-ray absorptiometry
- Single photon absorptiometry

---

dense, relatively little energy passes through. Bones that are weak, however, let a lot of rays slip through.

In young women, it's relatively easy to take bone readings directly from the spine. As women age, however, spinal bone density tests aren't as efficient. After age 65, the readings may be taken at the hips or wrists instead of the spine.

The National Osteoporosis Foundation recommends that women have bone density tests if they:

- Have low estrogen levels
- Show signs of vertebral abnormalities
- Have been found to have reduced bone mass on X-rays
- Are undergoing long-term treatment with corticosteroids
- Have a hormonal condition called hyperparathyroidism

Bone density tests aren't used very often, although many doctors believe they'll eventually become a standard test for measuring women's health. They usually cost about $800 to $900.

SPECIALISTS FOR BACK PAIN

Back pain is second only to the common cold as a reason Americans see their doctors. Not surprisingly, many doctors—as well as physical therapists, chiropractors, and other health professionals—are intimately familiar with back problems and their causes and solutions. (To learn about "alternative" forms of back care, see chapter 8.)

The place to begin, of course, is with your family doctor. Most back problems aren't particularly serious or complicated, and he will be able to advise you as to the proper course of treatment. Usually, this involves nothing more complicated than taking it easy for a few days and taking aspirin or a similar drug for pain and swelling.

Back problems that are more serious, however, may need to be treated by a specialist.

When to See a Specialist

Back pain is confusing because minor problems can be very painful while more serious problems may not be painful at all. You probably need to see a specialist when back pain is severe and doesn't go away within four to six weeks of treatment by your family doctor. Of course, your doctor may send you to a specialist much sooner if he suspects that something serious is going on.

You should also feel comfortable asking your doctor to refer you to a specialist—either because you want a second opinion or because you feel that more could be done for your problem.

Some back problems always require a specialist's care. If you're having pain or numbness in your legs or buttocks or you've lost bowel or bladder control, it could be an emergency and you should see a specialist right away.

There are many back pain specialists to choose from. Here are the ones you're most likely to see.

Neurologists

Your back is home not only to the spine and spinal cord but also to a variety of nerves that control strength and sensation in many parts of your body. As a result, back pain is often a shorthand way of referring to nerve pain.

A neurologist is a physician who specializes in the diagnosis and nonsurgical treatment of muscular and nervous system conditions, including problems affecting the back. Neurologists use a variety of sophisticated tests to check your reflexes, strength, and sensations. Problems such as a herniated disk and spinal stenosis are often diagnosed by a neurologist.

Neurosurgeons

Like neurologists, neurosurgeons are trained to recognize and treat muscular and nerve problems. They're also the hands-on experts. If you have a pinched nerve—due to a herniated disk, for example—a neurosurgeon may be the one who goes in and fixes it.

Orthopedic Surgeons

Any condition affecting the structures of your body—from your bones and joints to your muscles, ligaments, and tendons—is the province of orthopedic surgeons. They're quite comfortable handling nerve problems as well.

Orthopedic surgeons do more than just cut, however. They also discuss other treatments for back pain, such as braces, physical therapy, and home care.

Osteopathic Physicians

Unlike medical doctors, osteopathic doctors don't have M. D.'s after their names. (They're called D. O.'s.) They also undergo slightly different training than medical doctors. Osteopathic physicians are experts in bone and muscle problems and are more likely than M. D.'s to recommend hands-on care, such as spinal manipulation, for back pain.

Apart from this, their training is very similar to that received by medical doctors, and they specialize in the same areas, including neurology and surgery.

Physiatrists

Long-term back problems are never resolved overnight. They often require months or years of care—everything from physical therapy to regular exercise. Physiatrists are experts in this type of care. Their specialty is physical rehabilitation—not only for people with back pain but also for people with conditions such as strokes and brain injuries.

They are expert at the diagnosis and treatment of problems with the soft tissues of the lower back.

Physiatrists are very good at using nondrug therapies for easing back pain. (Of course, they prescribe drugs when necessary.) Just as important, they're good at finding ways to prevent it in the future. For people with back pain, physiatrists often design a comprehensive rehabilitation program. This usually includes things such as exercise, hot and cold packs, and sometimes transcutaneous electrical nerve stimulation, or TENS, to ease muscle pain. They also stress education and proper body mechanics—teaching people ways to strengthen their backs and to treat them more kindly in the future.

Occupational Therapists

Like any machine, your body is most efficient when it's used in the proper ways. In medicine, this is known as the science of ergonomics. Occupational therapists are well trained in ergonomics. They can teach you how to use your body—for sitting, standing, lifting, and any other kind of movement—in ways that won't be harmful for your back. Occupational therapists aren't doctors, however, and they can't prescribe drugs. They're often affiliated with hospital rehabilitation centers.

Physical Therapists

When you wrench your back on the soccer field or are recovering from surgery, there's a good chance your doctor will refer you to a physical therapist. Physical therapists aren't doctors, but they have specialized training in helping the body recover from injuries. They utilize everything from exercise and ultrasound to massage and electrical stimulation to help you get better. Like occupational therapists, they'll also show you ways to keep your back healthy in the future.

Exercise Physiologists

When your back is weak and out of shape, you may want to see an exercise physiologist. These aren't doctors, but they understand the body and will help you design an exercise program to improve muscle flexibility and strength. Exercise physiologists are often affiliated with hospitals and health centers, as well as health clubs.

Chiropractors

For years, many Americans have been confused about chiropractors, and for good reason. A number of studies have shown that people with back pain are more likely to be satisfied when they see a chiropractor than when they see a primary care provider (such as a family physician or an internist)—even though chiropractors sometimes charge more!

And yet the history of chiropractic care is an unusual one. Many older chiropractors believed that spinal misalignments, called subluxations, were responsible not only for back problems but for all diseases, including heart disease and diabetes.

Most chiropractors today have moved away from their traditional roots and are much closer to mainstream medical thought and practice. But they still believe that using hands-on care to manipulate the spine can be very helpful—not necessarily for heart disease, but certainly for problems such as back pain.

Chiropractors don't depend only on spinal adjustments, of course. They also use things such as massage, electrical stimulation, hot and cold packs, and exercise—the same techniques used by medical doctors.

The combination appears to be effective. One study found that people with acute back pain improved just as fast whether they saw a primary care doctor, a chiropractor, or an orthopedic surgeon. But here's the interesting part: Those who visited chiropractors were happier with the treatment they received.

More and more doctors now believe that seeing a chiropractor is a reasonable choice for simple back pain. In fact, the Agency for Health Care Policy and Research agrees that spinal manipulation is reasonable for low back pain during the first month of symptoms.

There are a few advantages to seeing a chiropractor. Chiropractors will often see their patients more frequently than medical doctors do. For similar episodes of back pain, people will visit their regular doctors about 3 times, compared with 10 visits to chiropractors. That's a lot of expert attention (often more than is really needed, some doctors feel). Many chiropractors either work with doctors or refer patients to doctors when they think it's necessary.

There are limits to what chiropractors can do, of course. They aren't medical doctors. They can order X-rays, but they can't prescribe medicine or perform surgery. They're not as well trained as doctors in handling serious back problems. That's why it's important to get your doctor's okay before seeing a chiropractor.

It is particularly important that herniated disks, vertebral fractures, and cancer not be treated with chiropractic, which can make these conditions worse. Also, it's best to avoid chiropractors who want to take full-body X-rays or who aggressively push dietary supplements.

Standard Treatments for Back Pain

Painful as they are, most back problems really aren't very serious. Although pulling a muscle or spraining a ligament can make you feel as though you've hauled a ton of bricks, the pain doesn't usually last long. Even degenerative changes to the spine, which naturally occur over time and cause wear and tear on the vertebrae and disks, are generally easy to manage. However, it is important to treat some back problems before they become less manageable and more painful.

The usual treatment for nearly all back pain—most doctors can recite it in their sleep—is to take it easy for a few days, take over-the-counter medications for pain, apply ice and heat, and start doing stretching exercises as soon as you feel up to it. It's simple, and it works—at least, it works for most people most of the time.

As recently as 10 years ago, doctors often prescribed powerful drugs and strict bed rest—as long as two weeks in some cases—for people with back pain. But they've since found that this approach isn't usually necessary. Even a potentially serious problem, such as a herniated disk, often gets better on its own within a few weeks or even a few days. Up to 90 percent of all back problems are entirely better in six to eight weeks.

Of course, once you've had one episode of back pain, there's a very good chance you'll have another. That's why most back care plans include a prescription for exercise. Aerobics is good. So are swimming, walking, and lifting weights. Anything you can do to strengthen muscles in your back, abdomen, and elsewhere in your body will go a long way toward preventing back pain in the future. Proper body mechanics—learning how to bend and to properly use your lower back—are also very important to ensure that you don't reinjure yourself.

Sometimes, of course, back pain goes on and on. That's when your doctor will recommend more intense kinds of treatments, such as physical therapy, wearing a back brace, or getting occasional chiropractic care. It's only as a last resort that doctors trot out the strong stuff, such as prescription drugs or expensive medical tests.

THE BEST SIMPLE TREATMENTS

The vast majority of backaches don't require expensive tests (or doctor visits). What they do need is time, along with some of the following:

- One to two days of bed rest
- Regular applications of ice and heat
- Over-the-counter medications
- Regular exercise to prevent recurrence
- Proper posture and body mechanics with instruction on bending and lifting
- Spinal manipulation by a chiropractor or physician, if recommended
- A back brace for a short period

Fortunately, it doesn't usually come to that. The simplest treatments are often the most effective.

THE GOVERNMENT GUIDELINES

To bring some consistency to the world of back pain—and also to separate the wheat from the chaff—the Agency for Health Care Policy and Research (AHCPR) has issued official guidelines. The agency's goal is to determine which strategies really work on back pain and which may be a waste of your time and money. (See "Lower Back Treatment Basics," on page 100.)

This isn't to say that every strategy not endorsed by the agency is necessarily worthless. In fact, there may be dozens of remedies for back pain that weren't even considered in drawing up the guidelines, or that had not been studied enough for the agency to feel confident in giving them either a thumbs-up or a thumbs-down.

One common treatment that "failed" the government guidelines is transcutaneous electrical nerve stimulation (TENS), despite the fact that it does appear to help some people. The agency also declined to recommend lumbar corsets (except when they're used as a preventive measure), back machines, and spinal traction. Prolonged bed rest also was rejected—a position most doctors today heartily agree with.

Keep in mind that the agency's guidelines are just that—guidelines, not hard and fast rules. If you've discovered some "trick" for managing back pain that clearly helps you but that isn't endorsed by the guidelines, don't quit. After all, your own back, and not some official summary, should have the last word. As long as it works and you and your doctor feel it isn't harmful, keep it up!

BED REST

It's common sense, but hardly anyone ever heeds it. When you hurt your back—while shoveling snow, for example—you know better than to keep going and finish the walk. But that's exactly what many people do: They grit their teeth and ignore the pain until they've finished whatever it is they set out to do. By that time, of course, their backs have flat-out had enough. So instead of one day in pain, they may be laid up for a week or more.

Listen to your body. When you feel back pain coming on, take a break. Slip off your shoes. Put on some relaxing music and lie down for 20 to 30 minutes. In some cases, that's all you'll need for your back to feel better.

But before you get up, move your back a little. How does it feel? At this point, you're the only one who can tell if it's just a minor twinge or if you've really wrenched something. If it hurts—really hurts—there's a good chance you've sprained a ligament or pulled a muscle. That's not going to get better in a half-hour. What you probably need is to take it easy for a day or two. Yes, it's inconvenient. Yes, you're a busy person. But how much time are you going to save if you rush things—and instead of a day in bed you end up horizontal for a week?

Rest is even more important if you have disk problems. (Telltale signs of disk trouble include shooting pain down one of your buttocks and legs and possibly a history of chronic back pain.) Even though a herniated disk always requires a doctor's care, simple bed rest and some physical therapy exercises will usually take care of it. Of course, unlike a strain or sprain, a herniated disk can keep you in bed, off and on, for up to several weeks.

Why is lying down so helpful for back pain? The reason is simple. When you lie down, you take almost all the weight off your spine. Without the constant pressure of hauling you around, your spine has a chance to heal.

Different people have different "positions of comfort." Most folks find that curling up in a fetal position with a pillow tucked between the knees is best for the back. Lying on your back with your knees slightly bent is also good, although holding your knees up for a long time can get tiring (slipping a pillow or two underneath your knees will help). You can try lying flat on your stomach, but you probably won't like it—it puts too much pressure on the spine.

Here's the interesting thing about bed rest. Some rest, for two to five days, may be good. Too much can make you worse. For one thing, lying in bed can cause your muscles to weaken and get stiff. In addition, prolonged bed rest can lead to depression, and that makes it even harder to get up later on. Being more active, on the other hand, promotes bone strength and also increases your levels of endorphins—chemicals produced by your brain that relieve pain and increase feelings of well-being.

In one study, researchers followed two groups of people with lower back pain. People in one group resumed their normal activities as soon as they felt able to do so. Those in the other group were given bed rest. Within a week, 20 percent of the active group hadn't yet returned to work. In the bed rest group, however, 41 percent hadn't returned to work. And after three months, folks in the bed rest group had taken an average of more than nine sick days. Those in the active group? They took a little less than five sick days. Up and at 'em after reasonable rest seems the best way to go.

ICE THERAPY

Cold doesn't feel as soothing as warmth. But in the immediate aftermath of a back injury, it's a lot more effective.

Applying cold packs—you can make your own by putting ice in a plastic bag and wrapping the bag in a washcloth or towel—eases back pain in several ways. For one thing, cold numbs the area, making the pain less intense. More important, it causes blood vessels to constrict, thus reducing blood flow to the area. This helps prevent swelling, which can dramatically reduce the pain you'll feel later on.

Doctors recommend applying cold to the painful area for 15 minutes at a time. If you're truly dedicated, it's a good idea to repeat the process once an hour for two days after the injury. At the very least, you should do it every few hours throughout the day.

Don't leave the cold on for too long, however, because it can damage your skin. When your skin starts getting numb, it's time to remove the ice, even if the 15 minutes isn't up.

HEAT THERAPY

While cold helps prevent swelling soon after an injury, heat is an excellent follow-up treatment. Applying heat warms the area, which helps relax the muscles. It will also increase blood flow, which speeds healing and eases stiffness.

You can buy commercial hot packs, but hot water bottles (or hot baths and showers) work just as well. The idea is to keep the area warm. Unlike cold therapy, heat therapy won't damage the skin. It's safe to apply heat for as long or as often as you want, as long as it's not too hot and it seems to help. (If you have diabetes or diminished skin sensation for any reason, however, never use extreme heat.)

If you belong to a gym, this would be a good time to try out the steam room or whirlpool or to go for a swim in the pool. The combination of heat and gentle exercise is ideal for relieving back pain and stiffness.

MEDICATIONS FOR BACK PAIN

There are dozens of over-the-counter and prescription pills that are commonly used for back pain. Most of them, however, fall into a few main categories.

- ◆ Over-the-counter pain relievers
- ◆ Narcotics such as codeine and morphine
- ◆ Muscle relaxants
- ◆ Antidepressants

PAIN MEDICATIONS

There's no lack of over-the-counter (OTC) remedies for backache. In fact, you may find that the number of choices—everything from aspirin (buffered or time-release, tablets or caplets) to ibuprofen and acetaminophen—is almost overwhelming.

For pain, it really doesn't matter what kind of OTC medicine you buy. We'll talk about these drugs in more detail in just a bit. For now, we'll just say they're about equally effective for pain. However, for the inflammation that often accompanies back pain, you'll want to buy aspirin, ibuprofen, or a similar drug. Acetaminophen (such as Tylenol) has little effect on inflammation.

Be sure to take these medications with food, without alcohol, and use them on a schedule (three times a day). Stop taking them if you develop indigestion or any other stomach problems.

When OTC medications don't work, your doctor may give you a prescription for more powerful drugs. These are often similar to aspirin in that they relieve pain and inflammation. They're stronger, however, and they occasionally cause side effects that may be troublesome, such as more severe stomach irritation and nausea. As a result, doctors usually advise using them only when OTC drugs don't help.

For the worst kinds of pain, your doctor may give you a prescription for narcotics (such as codeine), muscle relaxants, or even antidepressants. These drugs can be very helpful, but because of the risk of side effects—and, in the case of narcotics, the risk of addiction—they're always a last resort.

Over-the-Counter Medications

Aspirin is one of the oldest, least expensive medications you can buy. And despite decades (and billions of dollars) of research into a variety of other medications, it's still hard to beat for back pain.

These days, of course, there are many other OTC pills for pain, and more are being developed all the time. For now, we'll focus on aspirin, ibuprofen, and ketoprofen. (Acetaminophen acts somewhat differently, so we'll discuss it separately.) These drugs are known as nonsteroidal anti-inflammatory drugs (NSAIDs). Simply put, they not only relieve pain but also help stop swelling. They're considered some of the best drugs for stopping back pain.

Aspirin and other NSAIDs work by blocking the production of hormone-like compounds in the body known as prostaglandins. Prostaglandins cause swelling and also help to send pain impulses to the brain. When you block the prostaglandins, you block some of the discomfort as well.

No single NSAID has been found to work better than any other in relieving back pain. That said, people do tend to respond differently to these drugs. The only rule is to find the one that works best for you, while causing the fewest side effects.

Side effects can definitely be a concern. All these drugs can be hard on the stomach, with aspirin being the worst offender. (Ibuprofen, such as Motrin, generally causes fewer stomach problems.) To avoid stomach upset, doctors advise taking these medications along with food. In addition, you may want to try drugs that are enteric-coated: They have a tough layer that prevents the medicine from being released in the stomach. Instead, it passes through the stomach and dissolves in the intestines.

Another difficulty with NSAIDs is that they reduce the blood's ability to clot. So they can be a problem for women who are menstruating or for people who have any sort of bleeding disorder or who are going to have surgery.

Unlike NSAIDs, acetaminophen rarely causes side effects and is a good choice for stopping pain. Unfortunately, it doesn't stop inflammation, so it's not always as effective for every kind of back pain. You should not take more than 4,000 milligrams per day of acetaminophen and, as is true for all drugs, it should not be taken with alcohol, as this can cause liver damage.

Narcotics

Some people, because of allergies or side effects, can't take aspirin or aspirin-like drugs. What's more, some types of back pain simply are too severe for OTC help. It's the difference between "ouch" and real agony. That's when your doctor may write you a prescription for a drug such as codeine. Called narcotics, these medications work by reducing your brain's sensitivity to pain.

In some ways, narcotics are the gold standard for stopping pain—they're extremely effective. (Some brands also have aspirin or acetaminophen as ingredients because these make the narcotics work even better.) The problem, of course, is that narcotics can make you feel dopey and tired. They can also cause constipation. What's more, they may cause addiction in some people.

Doctors tend to prescribe narcotics for the first week following a back injury, when the pain is most severe. There's little risk of addiction in that early, acute period. After that, it's better to switch to milder (and safer) OTC drugs.

Muscle Relaxants

One reason back injuries are so painful is that the muscles, in an attempt to protect themselves, sometimes contract into hard, painful little knots called spasms. In some cases, the muscle spasms are more painful than the back injury itself.

To help your muscles relax and break the grip of spasms, doctors sometimes prescribe muscle relaxants. As with narcotics, they're normally used in the first week following an injury or a flare-up, when pain is at its peak.

Despite their name, muscle relaxants don't directly affect the muscles. What they do is depress the central nervous system, which in turn causes muscles to relax. Muscle relaxants can also help you sleep at night—which, when you have back pain, is no small favor.

Like narcotics, muscle relaxants cause side effects that can limit their use. They often make people feel drowsy and dizzy. They can also cause headache, a dry mouth, and nausea. And the side effects are often worse in older people, so dosages may need adjusting.

Antidepressants

They're not the first choice for back pain. But when other medications fail, antidepressants can be very helpful. These drugs work by increasing levels of serotonin and other feel-good chemicals in the brain. When levels of these chemicals rise, pain sensations may be reduced.

What's more, antidepressants can improve your mood and help you sleep. They can relieve the persistent pain of some long-lasting (and hard to treat) conditions such as fibromyalgia. And in some cases, tricyclic antidepressants such as amitriptyline hydrochloride (Elavil) are helpful against nerve pain. When these antidepressants are used for pain relief, they're usually given in much lower doses than those needed to treat depression.

Because they're given in low doses, serious side effects aren't often a problem. Some people, however, experience unpleasant sensations such as drowsiness, a dry mouth, constipation, or sensitivity to sunlight.

PHYSICAL THERAPY AND EXERCISE

When you're recovering from a serious bout of back pain, or when home treatments simply aren't working, your doctor may recommend that you see someone who specializes in making the body strong again. Physical therapists aren't doctors, but they're extremely knowledgeable about how the body works and what it needs to recover.

Physical therapists use a wide range of techniques, from massage, hydrotherapy (water treatments), and transcutaneous electrical nerve stimulation to ultrasound and customized exercise programs. But despite the range of treatments, the goal of each is similar: to relieve pain and make you stronger without resorting to medications or surgery.

There's solid scientific evidence that physical therapy works. Techniques such as massage, hydrotherapy, and ultrasound increase the flow of blood and oxygen to painful muscles in your back. This generates heat in the muscles, giving soothing relief.

More importantly, physical therapy can help get you started on a safe exercise plan that's tailored to your condition and circumstances. As you start getting stronger and more flexible, the risk of future episodes of back pain can drop dramatically.

Posture and Body Mechanics

Education about how to move and how to lift safely can be one of the most important factors in avoiding future episodes of low back pain. Proper sitting posture, too, and correct technique for use of your lower back will also help to prevent future problems.

Aerobic, Flexibility, and Strengthening Exercises

The only thing better for your back than routine exercise is a combination of exercises. Doctors often advise people with back pain to take up aerobic, flexibility, and strengthening exercises. Individually, they're good. In combination, they can strengthen your whole body, keep you limber, make your bones stronger, and prevent recurrent attacks of pain.

You already know about the heart-and-lung workout you get with aerobic exercises such as swimming and the mobility-enhancing benefits of regular stretching. But what, exactly, are weight-bearing exercises?

For starters, forget the name "weight-bearing exercises." It's confusing. Instead, think walking. Lifting weights. Even dancing. Each of these activities requires your muscles to push against gravity—in other words, they're bearing weight. (In the case of walking, you're moving your own body weight—just try doing that with barbells!)

Weight-bearing exercises relieve back pain in several ways. They make muscles stronger, and better able to support the back and spine. What's more, research has shown that people who do weight-bearing exercises actually build more bone, which makes the vertebrae heavier and stronger.

This can be especially important for women because weight-bearing exercises can help reverse the bone-thinning effects of osteoporosis. In fact, there's some evidence that young women who exercise can "warehouse" bone, so they have more available as they get older. This can help reduce the risk of vertebral fractures, which are common in older women.

Weight-bearing exercises are also recommended for people who are taking powerful anti-inflammatory medications called corticosteroids, which essentially rob the body of bone-strengthening calcium.

To learn more about exercise and back pain, see chapter 7.

SPINAL MANIPULATION

Spinal manipulation has recently received the federal government's seal of approval for the short-term treatment of back pain. Performed by chiropractors, physiatrists, and osteopathic physicians, spinal manipulation involves adjusting joints and vertebrae in the back and neck to bring them into alignment.

It's not entirely clear why it works. In fact, there's scant scientific evidence to prove that it does work. However, a great many people with back pain swear by it, so it's certainly worth a try. The exception is if you have a herniated disk or another serious back problem that is causing nerve pain. In these situations, it's possible that spinal manipulation will make the problem worse instead of better.

LOWER BACK TREATMENT BASICS

The Agency for Health Care Policy and Research has issued guidelines for the treatment of acute lower back problems. Here's a quick summary.

Remember: Most people start to feel better soon!

**Over-the-counter medications
(for mild to moderate symptoms):**
- These include aspirin, ibuprofen, and acetaminophen.
- They have fewer side effects and are less expensive than prescription drugs.

**Prescription medications
(for more severe symptoms):**
- Some may cause drowsiness, so use caution when driving or operating heavy equipment.
- Other possible side effects include nausea, vomiting, and dizziness. If these occur, stop taking the medication and call your health care provider immediately.

Treatments to use alone or with medication:
- *Cold.* Apply a cold pack or ice to the painful area for 5 to 10 minutes at a time within the first 48 hours.
- *Heat.* Use a heating pad or hot shower or bath if symptoms last longer than 48 hours.
- *Spinal manipulation.* An experienced professional can manipulate the spine during the first month of lower back symptoms.

Other treatments:
These may provide short-term relief but have not been shown to speed recovery or prevent the recurrence of acute back problems. They may also be expensive.

- Acupuncture
- Back corsets
- Biofeedback
- Injections to the back
- Massage
- Traction
- Ultrasound
- Transcutaneous electrical nerve stimulation (TENS)

Bed rest:
- Limit to two or three days. Lying down can weaken muscles and prolong recovery time.
- If you must lie down, get up every few hours and walk around—even if you feel some discomfort.

Physical activity:
If the pain is severe, you should avoid:
- Heavy lifting
- Lifting when twisting, bending forward, or reaching
- Sitting for long periods

Returning to work:
- With your health care provider and employer, decide how much you are able to do safely.
- Increase your work activities gradually as your symptoms improve.
- Do only those things at work or at home that you are able to do comfortably.
- If your pain increases, tell your employer, coworkers, and family.
- Be clear about what you can and cannot do.

Back Schools

One of the reasons back pain is so hard to beat is that it has literally dozens of causes—from the way you sit or stand to the way you tie your shoes. It's easy to tell someone to "change your lifestyle." But it's not so easy to put into practice. That's where a back school can help.

Back schools, which were developed in Sweden by a physical therapist named Maryanne Zachrisson-Forsell, essentially offer a "back tech" degree for people in pain. The programs are usually offered by hospitals and YMCAs. They're directed by physical therapists under the supervision of physicians.

Back schools teach everyday, practical ways to keep your back strong—and to avoid the 1,001 things that can make it worse. Along with other folks with back pain, you'll learn exercises, how to sit and stand correctly, and how to lift without hurting yourself. You'll also learn tips for reducing stress and coping with setbacks.

Although there is no clear scientific evidence that back schools will prevent future episodes, there's no question that education is your best defense in avoiding them.

Transcutaneous Electrical Nerve Stimulation (TENS)

The spinal cord and nerves are essentially electrical conduits, sending signals—including pain signals—throughout your body. As it turns out, an effective way to fight pain's electricity is with more electricity.

Transcutaneous electrical nerve stimulation (TENS) is a therapy in which electrodes attached to the skin transmit a painless, low-voltage current. You feel a kind of strong tingling sensation. The current stimulates nerves, which is thought to "distract" the brain from noticing pain. (When the brain doesn't notice it, you don't notice it.) In addition, the current may stimulate production of the body's pain-killing endorphins.

TENS isn't a cure. The relief it provides is usually short-lived, and many experts feel it's not worth the bother. Still, a minority of people undergoing this treatment have found it to be effective comfort. It's worth asking your doctor if TENS might be right for you.

BRACES AND BELTS

Like girdles, back braces have gone in and out of fashion. At one time, they were all the rage in back pain circles. After a while, doctors began to consider them about as useful as whale-bone corsets and consigned them to the storage room. Today, however, they're back on the scene.

In one large study beginning in 1989, Home Depot employees in California whose jobs required them to lift or move heavy items were told to wear 8- to 10-inch-wide Lycra spandex back supports. Five years later, researchers were amazed when they looked at the results. The rate of lower back injuries had dropped by a remarkable one-third.

Doctors aren't sure if back belts prevent problems by supporting the back. They do believe, however, that the belts help remind people to do their bending and lifting more carefully. The belts are inexpensive and certainly worth a try. The trick, of course, is to not pick up more weight when you're wearing the belt than you would without it! And, remember to use proper body mechanics. (For more on proper lifting techniques, see chapter 6.)

TRACTION AND CORSETS

Fifteen years ago, a back problem might have sent you to the hospital, where you would have spent a few days or weeks harnessed to counterweights, or in traction. And when you walked out the door, you probably would have been wearing a corset to "hold the back in place."

For the most part, traction and corsets have gone the way of the horse-and-buggy. There's simply no evidence that they work. Plus, they're terribly uncomfortable.

As is typical with back pain, however, there are exceptions. Doctors occasionally recommend corsets for people who are recovering from surgery or whose back pain is severe enough without the corset that they can't perform even simple activities. And occasionally, therapists will use a brief course of traction, or autotraction, which is the weight of your own body, to reduce discomfort.

For the most part, however, both corsets and prolonged periods of traction should be viewed as medical curiosities rather than as practical treatments for back pain.

CHAPTER FIVE

When Surgery
May Be Necessary

Back pain isn't like appendicitis, when the first twinge means it's time to call a surgeon. The vast majority of back problems, including those that affect nerves, get better with time and home care—what doctors call conservative care. Only about 1 percent of people with back problems need surgery, and doctors are increasingly reluctant to operate until all other options have been explored.

Even when back pain is chronic—that is, it lasts longer than 12 weeks—doctors prefer to first try gentler, noninvasive treatments, such as bed rest, stretching exercises, and pain medications.

Yet certain types of back problems, especially those involving stubborn herniated disks or severe cases of spinal stenosis, may require surgery. In addition, there are some emergency situations when surgery is necessary, such as when there's pressure on the critical cauda equina bundle of nerves.

Even when surgery is required, it doesn't usually have to be done right away. There is time to get a second opinion and to weigh the options—the benefits you're likely to receive versus the possible risks of the surgery. And of course, you can take some time to see if more conservative, nonsurgical options can help.

WHEN YOU MAY NEED SURGERY

Most back surgery is elective—that is, you can do it now or later or even avoid it entirely. But some conditions almost always require surgery.

Emergency surgery is required when:
- There's an abscess in the spine (an epidural abscess).
- There's a spinal tumor.
- You have a serious nerve problem (such as cauda equina syndrome) with loss of bowel or bladder control.
- You have certain types of spinal fractures.

Elective surgery is an option when:
- You have sciatica caused by a herniated disk and the pain or loss of sensation has lasted for four to six weeks.
- You have persistent pain due to spinal stenosis or spondylolisthesis.
- You have severe spinal stenosis.
- You have chronic, persistent, neck or lower back pain.
- You have certain spinal deformities.
- You have persistent arm or leg nerve pain.
- You have persistent spinal infection.
- You have certain types of tumor.

Ultimately, having surgery is a very individual choice. Now let's take a look at when surgery is likely to be called for, what kind of conservative care may be tried first, and what to expect if you do undergo an operation.

SURGERY FOR A HERNIATED DISK: DISKECTOMY

The spinal disks are gel-filled pads that sit between vertebrae in the spine. When a disk ruptures (herniates), the gel inside may ooze out and press against nearby nerves, causing excruciating pain. Sometimes the pain goes away on its own. When it doesn't, you may need surgery to remove all or portions of the damaged disk. The operation to remove a disk is called a diskectomy.

About 200,000 diskectomies are performed in the United States every year. Surgeons get a lot of practice doing them, and serious complications are rare. According to some estimates, however, 5 to 15 percent of these procedures don't work as well as they might, and then further operations are necessary.

Nonsurgical Treatment

Having a herniated disk doesn't mean you need surgery. (Disks that rupture high in the spine are more likely to require surgery than those in the lumbar, or lower back, area.) In general, about 90 percent of people with ruptured disks get better with home care. This is because it's not the damaged disk itself that causes serious pain. Rather, the pain occurs when portions of the disk begin pressing on nerves. You can often relieve nerve pain by resting and taking anti-inflammatory medications. Then the damaged disk is less of a problem.

Even when home care doesn't help, there are other options besides surgery. Doctors sometimes inject cortisone (an anti-inflammatory steroid) or procaine (an anesthetic) into the ruptured disk. These injections are somewhat risky, and there's no scientific evidence that they will work for all people. In some cases, however, they may reduce pain and swelling and allow the nerve to heal on its own.

Yet another nonsurgical option is for the doctor to inject an anti-inflammatory steroid such as cortisone into the base of the spine or neck rather than directly into the disk. This may help relieve nerve pain for people with disk disease as well as for those with spinal stenosis. For some people with nerve pain, this procedure may be worth considering when nonsteroidal anti-inflammatory medications have failed, or are not an option due to side effects.

A CHEMICAL ALTERNATIVE

The next time you pick up a bottle of meat tenderizer, read the label. It probably contains a substance similar to chymopapain, a naturally occurring enzyme derived from the papaya fruit. Surgeons have discovered that the same stuff that tenderizes a tough flank steak may be used to treat a herniated disk as well.

With a procedure called chemonucleolysis, chymopapain is injected into a herniated spinal disk. It literally tenderizes the disk, breaking down the gel-like material and relieving painful pressure on the nerve.

This procedure is controversial and has fallen in and out of favor over the years. When it's successful, it can relieve the pain of a herniated disk without the need for surgery. But about 1 percent of patients will have a dangerous—and potentially fatal—allergic reaction to chymopapain. (This has become much less of a risk in recent years, however, as special tests can now determine whether you are allergic to the enzyme.) And, if the needle is misdirected, nerve damage could result. Finally, the procedure is hardly painless. Some people will have pain and muscle spasms for several days after the treatment.

When It's Time for Surgery

Surgery is a last resort, and your doctor will do everything possible to avoid it. But some herniated disks simply won't get better with conservative treatment. If the nerve damage is causing a loss of bowel or bladder control, severe pain that isn't getting better (or is actually getting worse), or persistent weakness in the muscles, you're probably going to need surgery.

The Operation

Surgery for a herniated disk is usually done while you are under general anesthesia. Once your surgeon has exposed the spinal area, he'll make an incision, or cut, into the damaged disk and remove the gel-like material. (It may be necessary to remove part of a vertebra in order to reach the damaged disk.) Once the gel has been removed, there's no more pressure on the nerve. It can begin healing on its own.

In addition, your surgeon may decide to use bone grafts to fuse, or join, two adjoining vertebrae. This gives more stability and strength to the spine, which can help prevent future problems from occurring. Most of the time, however, spinal fusion isn't required for disk herniation.

Surgery for a herniated spinal disk is quite straightforward, and complications are rare. In some cases, however, there may be a tear of the dura mater—the membrane that protects the spinal cord. There's also a slight risk that nerves will be damaged during the operation.

Other Types of Surgery

Surgeons are constantly exploring other, less invasive (and less painful) approaches to disk surgery. Some of these techniques show great promise. In fact, some of the newer techniques for disk surgery can even be done under local anesthetic. Some people have the operation and go home the same day.

One surgical option is called microdiskectomy. Unlike traditional disk operations, which require a large incision, microdiskectomy can be done through a small (1- to $1\frac{1}{2}$-inch) incision. The smaller incision means less trauma during the operation and faster recovery afterward.

Another option is called percutaneous arthroscopic diskectomy. This doesn't require an incision at all. Instead, the surgeon—guided by X-rays—inserts a small probe through the skin and uses it to remove the stray material that's protruding from the damaged disk.

Finally, some surgeons have explored a type of surgery called laser diskectomy. Rather than mechanically removing the damaged disk material, the surgeon uses a laser to burn out the inside of the disk. So far, this procedure doesn't appear to work any better than conventional disk surgery.

Recuperation

Since a traditional diskectomy often requires a larger incision, it may take several weeks before your back is really strong again. You can expect to spend one to two days in the hospital. Once you're home, the disk (and the irritation around the nerve) will slowly begin to heal. Most people are able to return to work six to eight weeks after the operation. If you've had more than one operation, however, your recovery time may be quite a bit longer, and the results may not be as satisfactory.

Expected Results

Surgery for herniated disks can be very successful. Between 75 and 95 percent of people who undergo diskectomies will be completely free of sciatic nerve pain, and about 15 percent will obtain at least partial relief. About 70 percent will be free of back pain as well as pain from the injured nerve.

However, doctors have found that years later most people are likely to wind up with the same amount of relief whether they have surgery or use more conservative treatments. So even though surgery may be essential to relieve severe pain and is important for preventing and treating nerve damage, it isn't necessary for most people.

WHEN YOU MAY NEED SURGERY FOR A HERNIATED DISK

For most herniated disks, surgery is considered elective—that is, you can choose whether or not to undergo the procedure. Sometimes, however, it's the only choice. You're going to need surgery when:

- You've lost control of your bowels or bladder. (This is an emergency—seek medical help immediately.)
- You have persistent nerve pain that isn't relieved by rest.
- Your muscles are growing progressively weaker.
- You're having repeated attacks of severe sciatica.

SURGERY FOR VERTEBRAL COMPRESSION FRACTURES: SPINAL FUSION

The vertebrae in your spine are normally locked into place with a series of joints and stretchy ligaments. This is what makes the spinal column flexible yet strong.

But when vertebrae are fractured—due to damage from an accident or another traumatic injury, for example—the entire spine may be weakened. To keep the spine strong, surgeons sometimes do spinal fusion, in which two or more adjoining vertebrae are permanently locked together with bone grafts. Spinal fusion is sometimes done following diskectomies as well. (For more on fusion surgery for vertebral compression fractures resulting from osteoporosis, see chapter 2.)

Nonsurgical Treatment

The pain caused by fractured vertebrae is often due to inflammation. For most folks, simple home remedies such as bed rest and over-the-counter medications are all that are needed. In more serious cases, a back brace may help, along with remedies such as applying ice or hot packs. In addition, your doctor may recommend drugs to slow the bone loss that's actually causing the problem. In most cases, the bone will heal in about 8 to 12 weeks.

When It's Time for Surgery

As with many back problems, the guidelines for surgery are fairly straightforward: When you're in severe pain or the pain doesn't go away (or it does go away but often comes back), you may need surgery to repair the damage.

The Operation

Spinal fusion is done under general anesthetic, so you can plan on spending several days in the hospital. It also currently requires at least two incisions—one in the spinal area and another in the pelvis, from which the bone grafts will be "harvested."

During the procedure, your surgeon will take bone from your pelvis and place, or graft, it in the area of the damaged vertebrae. Bone is living tissue and, over time, it will begin to grow. Eventually, the growing bone will fuse the damaged vertebrae together, making them stronger and stabilizing your spine. In some cases, the surgeon will also implant a metal fixation device, such as a plate or screw, to enhance bone healing. This may be done in some operations for arm and leg fractures as well. (To learn about new techniques that are being pioneered for spinal fusion and fractured vertebrae, see chapter 9.)

Recuperation

You don't recover from spinal fusion surgery overnight. Although you'll probably be able to get out of bed two or three days after the surgery, the bone grafts will require about six months to take permanent hold. During that time the spine must be kept immobile. Most people wear back braces—not all the time, but a lot of the time—for 6 to 24 weeks after the procedure.

Expected Results

Spinal fusion is often necessary, and the results vary according to the severity of the condition. The surgery is successful in 60 to 85 percent of cases, studies show.

WHEN YOU MAY NEED SPINAL FUSION

Spinal fusion isn't a simple operation, so it's done only when pain is severe or when the spine is becoming dangerously unstable. Conditions that may require spinal fusion include:

- Herniated disks
- Vertebral fractures
- Spondylolisthesis
- Rheumatoid arthritis of the spine
- Severe scoliosis or kyphosis
- Tumors
- Some cases of spinal stenosis
- Some spinal infections

SURGERY FOR SPINAL STENOSIS: DECOMPRESSION SURGERY

Your spine isn't made up of solid bone. Running the entire length of the spinal column is the spinal canal, a hollow tube that contains the spinal cord and other nerves.

In people with spinal stenosis, the spinal canal becomes too narrow to comfortably house the spinal cord and other nerves. Over time, the "walls" of the spine may begin pressing on the spinal cord, causing pain and other symptoms. To relieve the pressure, doctors often recommend decompression surgery, which enlarges the spinal canal, or increases the size of openings in the vertebrae where the nerves leave the spine. Spinal fusion may also be necessary.

Nonsurgical Treatment

Spinal stenosis doesn't always cause serious symptoms. For mild pain, over-the-counter medications may be helpful. Losing weight and doing stretching or flexion exercises can also help ease the discomfort.

In more serious cases, doctors sometimes inject pain medications or anti-inflammatory steroids into the spinal area. If you have Paget's disease, a condition in which bones in the spine get thick and "crumbly," your doctor may prescribe medications that help make your bones stronger and more compact, so they're less likely to press on nearby nerves.

When It's Time for Surgery

Any time there's pressure on a nerve, there's a risk of serious symptoms. Some people with spinal stenosis lose control of their bowels or bladder. What's more, the constant pressure can be extraordinarily painful. And when pain is that persistent, your legs may weaken, which can even limit your ability to walk. When conservative care isn't helping, you're probably going to need surgery to widen the canal and give the spinal cord and nerves more room to "breathe."

The Operation

The principle of decompression surgery is quite simple: Removing excess bone will quickly reduce pressure on the nerves and relieve pain.

During the operation, which is done under general anesthesia, your surgeon will open up the spinal canal in the areas where narrowing has occurred. Using a variety of instruments, your surgeon will essentially cut away bone, enlarging the spinal canal and the openings where the nerves leave the spine. In addition, he may need to remove ligaments or other types of fibrous tissue that may be putting pressure on the nerves.

One problem with this procedure is that removing bone from the spinal canal can weaken its bony supports. If the spine then seems too rickety, your surgeon may also fuse two or more vertebrae together, which will make the spine stronger.

Recuperation

You can plan on spending four to seven days in the hospital following decompression surgery. It's an "aggressive" operation, so you can expect to be considerably sore afterward. Most people start walking—with some help from a walker—a day or two after the surgery. In addition, you'll probably need to use a cane for 6 to 12 weeks, or until you can comfortably walk on your own.

If you have a spinal fusion during the operation, your recovery will be slower. You'll probably be required to wear a back brace for about three months afterward. And if you smoke cigarettes, you'll need to stop to improve bone healing during the recovery period.

Expected Results

Surgeons say that if decompression surgery is indicated, the results are usually excellent. This is especially true when the spinal narrowing is limited to one or two places. Leg pain, a major problem in spinal stenosis, is improved or eliminated in 70 to 85 percent of people who have the operation.

One study that compared surgical and nonsurgical treatments for spinal stenosis found that people who had surgery for spinal stenosis were more satisfied with their progress than those who opted for nonsurgical treatments—this despite the fact that those in the surgical group had more severe problems to begin with.

Decompression surgery usually is quite safe. But because many people who have the operation are elderly and also suffer from other conditions, such as arthritis or heart disease, there may be other complications that are not directly related to the surgery.

CHAPTER SIX

Staying Healthy:
How to Prevent Future
Episodes of Back Pain

Imagine that about once a month, year in and year out, someone came up behind you and, for no reason whatsoever, gave you a thump with a two-by-four. Not a little love tap, either, but a roundhouse wallop that took your breath away. After a while, chances are you wouldn't exactly look forward to getting out of bed in the mornings.

Hard to imagine? Not for people with bad backs. They know that sooner or later they're going to get walloped—not every month, maybe, but way too often. Back pain is rarely a one-time thing. If you've had one episode of back pain, there's a better than 50-50 chance that you'll have another within two years. And that's if you're lucky. For some people, back attacks—along with muscle spasms, stiffness, and sundry other painful symptoms—strike with alarming frequency.

But it doesn't have to be this way. Doctors have found that a lot of the simple choices you make every day—having a fast-food (and high-fat) meal instead of a beans-and-greens salad, for example, or watching TV instead of taking a walk—can have a direct impact on your back. You might not think that a healthy lifestyle would make that much difference, but it does.

People who are overweight, for instance, often have back pain because the spine and muscles have to work harder to carry the extra pounds around. Have you been watching more TV lately? The time you spend sitting creates enormous stress on your lower back, increasing the risk of disk damage.

Even simple things such as not getting enough calcium in your diet can create serious problems later on. In fact, having a glass or two of low-fat milk a day—along with all the calcium it contains—can vastly reduce your risk of osteoporosis, one of the leading causes of vertebral fractures and other back problems.

Are you taking time to stop and smell the roses instead of worrying all the time? You should. "Unhealthy" emotions such as depression, anxiety, and stress can put your muscles in a perpetual state of red-alert tension, leading to sprains or strains.

In this chapter, we'll look at some very practical things you can do every day to make yourself healthier and to keep your back strong—everything from standing up a little straighter to choosing foods that won't hurt your back (or your waistline). No, these changes aren't always convenient. But in the scope of things, they're not that hard, either. And even if they were, think of the trade-off. Wouldn't you gladly swap a hamburger for a salad once or twice a week if you knew it would save you a week of bed rest? Take a walk in the evenings in exchange for giving up your pain pills? Practice a few minutes of meditation or positive thinking instead of canceling your vacation because your back hurts too much to get around?

There's no question that a healthy lifestyle can help prevent back problems. But even if you have a history of back pain, there are ways to take out the kinks—without using drugs or spending money for unnecessary visits to the doctor. There are a number of excellent products on the market that can help prevent back pain as well as help it retreat more quickly. Better yet, you can learn ways to use your back so that it doesn't get hurt in the first place. We'll even show you new ways to sleep that will help you wake up refreshed—and not be afraid to climb out of bed in the morning.

YOUR WEIGHT AND BACK PAIN

If a stranger walked up and told you to pick up a knapsack, fill it with rocks, and carry it around all day, you'd tell him where to park it. But millions of Americans are essentially doing this to themselves every day—not with rocks, of course, but with extra body weight.

Being overweight is one of the worst things for your back. Extra pounds cause problems in a number of different ways. Muscles that are overworked tire easily, leading to sprains or strains. Extra weight puts pressure on the spine, exaggerating its normal curve. This in turn is bad for your posture and terrible for your spinal disks: The combination of extra weight and unevenly distributed pressure can make disks much more likely to herniate or degenerate, causing arthritis, sciatica and other types of nerve pain.

Here's another way in which those extra pounds cause problems. As you already know, careful lifting is essential to protect your back. One of the requirements of careful lifting of heavy objects is keeping them close to your body, where the leverage is greater. But the simple truth is, when you're carrying extra weight around your middle, it becomes impossible to hold things close—you have to reach out farther with your arms. This throws off your center of gravity, putting tremendous strain on your lower back.

Losing weight is never easy, of course. But the tremendous benefits—more mobility, less back pain, and better overall health—make it worth the effort. What's the best way to begin?

Not with diets. They don't work, for the simple reason that it's nearly impossible for people to spend the rest of their lives totting up calories and worrying about every bite. A better strategy, doctors say, is not to eat less but to eat better. Here's what they advise.

Eliminate some of the fat from your diet. Many of the foods we like best, from ice cream to T-bone steaks, are very high in fat. The problem with fat is that it contains about twice as many calories as an equal serving of protein or carbohydrate. In other words, it's calorie-dense, which means you don't have to eat a lot of fat to see it on the scale the next morning.

Doctors recommend cutting the amount of fat in your diet to no more (and preferably less) than 30 percent of the total calories you take in. This isn't hard to do. In fact, you don't even have to give up your favorite foods. Simply eating them a little less often—by swapping that cheeseburger for a salad, for example—will go a long way toward keeping your fat intake at a healthy level.

Eat from the garden. You don't have to become a vegetarian to lose weight. But eating more vegetables—along with more fruits and grains—is still an essential part of any weight-loss plan. For one thing, these foods contain virtually no fat, which means you can eat a lot of them without worrying about your waistline. What's more, fruits, vegetables, and grains are high in dietary fiber. Fiber is unique because it absorbs tremendous amounts of water in your system. This means it fills you up and keeps you feeling satisfied longer than many richer—and more fattening—foods.

Savor your pleasures. One of the hardest things about trying to lose weight is that no one looks forward to giving up the foods they really enjoy, such as chocolate and ice cream. So don't give them up! When you have a taste for something sweet, have it. Enjoy. Just don't enjoy a big quantity, and don't enjoy it all the time.

This is really the key to losing weight. Don't try to starve yourself, and don't give up the pleasure you get from food. Nutritionists agree that all foods are "good" foods as long as you eat them only occasionally and in reasonable quantities. Besides, you're far more likely to stay motivated and to keep losing weight when you can look forward to life's little pleasures along the way.

A MINERAL FOR YOUR BACK

Your body uses calcium for all sorts of things. It is an electrolyte, meaning it carries an electrical charge that the body uses to transmit nerve signals and to control muscle movements. And of course, it's essential for bone strength.

When you don't get enough calcium in your diet, your body has to get the calcium it needs from somewhere—and your bones are a particularly rich source. If your intake of calcium remains low, your body "withdraws" more and more of this essential mineral from the bones, causing them to get thin and brittle—a condition called osteomalacia. Osteomalacia is the decreased mineralization of bones, which can result in osteoporosis, or decreased bone mass.

The most common cause of fractured vertebrae—what doctors call vertebral compression fractures—is osteoporosis, caused by low levels of calcium in the diet. This is especially true in women past menopause, when flagging estrogen causes calcium levels to decline.

Even though osteoporosis is one of the major causes of bone fractures, it's very easy to prevent. Here's how.

Pour a glass of milk. Along with yogurt and cheese, milk is one of the best sources of calcium you can find—and it's also fortified with vitamin D, which your body needs to help absorb the calcium. What's more, the calcium in dairy foods is much easier for the body to absorb than the calcium found in virtually any other food. (Low-fat and nonfat dairy foods are your healthiest bets.)

Eat green (and yellow). Leafy green vegetables such as broccoli, kale, and spinach, and yellow vegetables such as winter squash, are very good sources of calcium. They can't compete with dairy foods. But if you don't like milk or cheese, or if you simply want to get as much additional calcium in your diet as you can, they're excellent choices.

Open a can. For taste as well as nutrition, fresh foods should be your first choice. But when you're trying to take in extra calcium to protect your spine, you can't do much better than canned sardines. These tasty little fish contain soft bones, which are edible and very high in calcium. Another alternative is canned salmon, which contains ground soft salmon bones.

Drink some sunshine. Fortified juices are great calcium finds. Recently, many orange juice producers have begun offering orange juice with calcium next to the regular kinds.

Soak up some sunshine. Don't like milk enough to get your daily dose of vitamin D? Then spend 15 minutes, once a week, in the sun. Your body will produce vitamin D whenever sunshine caresses your skin—which is why D has been called the sunshine vitamin.

Consider supplements. If you simply can't get enough calcium in your diet—and for women in particular, getting enough calcium is always a challenge—you can't go wrong by taking calcium supplements. Daily supplements will help keep your calcium at healthy levels and are a very powerful remedy for preventing bone and back problems later on.

GOOD CALCIUM SOURCES

Calcium is essential for both men and women. But for women, the need is even more urgent. Doctors recommend that women past menopause get at least 1,500 milligrams of calcium a day. Unfortunately, government studies reveal that most women get only about 450 milligrams a day.

Many foods contain calcium. Here are some of the best sources.

Food	Calcium (mg)
Milk, 8 oz.	300
Yogurt, 8 oz.	275
Swiss cheese, 1 oz.	260
Sardines, 3½ oz.	250
Cottage cheese, 1 cup	210
Salmon, 3½ oz.	100

If you don't see yourself downing enough of these in a day, your doctor may suggest that you consider a calcium-rich supplement such as Tums or Oscal.

TAKE THE EDGE OFF STRESS

It's the classic chicken-or-egg conundrum. For years, doctors have noticed that people who have a lot of stress in their lives are much more likely to have back pain than folks who are more relaxed. Does this mean that stress causes back pain—or that people with back pain are naturally (and understandably) a little stressed?

Actually, it's probably a little of both. If you've had a bad day at the office lately, you know that even a moderate amount of stress can make you more sensitive to all kinds of things, including pain. In fact, doctors have found that people tend to experience pain more often (and more dramatically) when they are depressed or going through rough times than when they're feeling good.

The other side of the equation, of course, is that people with back pain feel less confident and less in control. It's hard for them to move. They can't do the things they like. They are, not surprisingly, under stress—and that makes the back pain worse.

It doesn't really matter which comes first—the stress or the pain. The important point is this: Anything you can do to reduce the amount of stress in your life—exercising, meditating, doing yoga, writing in a journal, or taking a film class once a week—is going to help your back.

As the writer Henry David Thoreau pointed out many years ago, simplifying your life is one of the best ways to achieve peace and tranquillity. We can't all retire to Walden Pond, of course. But there are many simple steps you can take to create a little more breathing space in your life. Here are a few ideas you may want to try.

Learn to delegate. When your back is hurting, you need help. This isn't a luxury—it's a necessity. So let the kids prepare dinner (and do the dishes afterward). Ask your colleagues to bring papers to your desk. Have your spouse do the driving for a few days. Anything you can do to make your life less stressed will pay off for your back.

Use the phone book. Even in hectic, modern America, good service is alive and well. There are a surprising number of businesses—from pharmacies to take-out Chinese restaurants—that still deliver. Take advantage of it now and then. Yes, it costs a bit more. But so what? Making your life a little less chaotic will do wonders for your stress level, and, ultimately, for your back. What's a better investment?

Form a car pool. Between ballet classes, Little League, and after-school activities, parents today do more driving than their parents ever dreamed of. This affects more than just your credit card. Doctors have found that driving is very hard on the back. What's more, the constant stress of being on time and "on-call" can wear you out.

See if you can form a car pool with some of the other parents in your neighborhood or at your kids' school. Car pools aren't always easy to set up, but they can save you a ton of anxiety and time. And remember, other parents will be just as eager as you are to reduce the drive time in their lives!

Obviously, these are just a few of the thousands of things you can try to make your life a little bit simpler. Take a few minutes to write down some of your own ideas, or check out your favorite bookstore for some of the new books on living simply. You owe it to yourself to live your life well—and you can't do it when you're running crazy all the time.

STOPPING STRESS FROM THE INSIDE OUT

It's not an exaggeration to say that stress is a tenacious adversary. It comes on slowly, creeping into your life along with all the tight deadlines, late bills, and family spats. By the time you're even aware of it, it has infiltrated your life—and your back is paying the price.

As we've seen, there are many simple lifestyle changes that can help reduce stress. Now we'll look at a few that aren't quite as simple—but can be very effective and well worth your time.

Biofeedback

Ever since Russian physiologist Ivan Pavlov trained his dogs to drool for food at the ring of a bell, doctors have known that many of the body's "automatic" functions—such as heart rate, blood pressure, muscle tension, and saliva-tion—can be changed when you put your mind to it. This is important because some of the things that cause back pain, such as muscle tension, are actually within your control.

Therapists use a technique called biofeedback to teach people to control their own bodies. In biofeedback, small electrode sensors are placed on the skin to measure things such as muscle tension. When you mentally relax—as a result of meditation, for example—the biofeedback machine tells you with an audible tone that your body is following suit.

By following these electronic cues, you can learn to consciously relax your back muscles. Once you get good at doing this, you won't need the machine anymore. You'll be able to relax your muscles at any time and in any place— even when you're standing in the checkout line.

Relaxation

We tend to think that relaxing is as natural as breathing. But in today's fast-paced world, it's anything but. That's why doctors often advise people with back problems to "work" at relaxing. That sounds funny, but once you've developed the skills, relaxing can substantially reduce stress—and, of course, much of your back pain.

Doctors aren't entirely sure why relaxation is so good for the back. But it's free, it doesn't take long, and many people with back pain swear by it. It's certainly worth a try.

There are many techniques for achieving deep, back-saving relaxation. Here are a few of the most effective.

Progressive relaxation. This is a technique in which you consciously tell all your muscles to relax. Here's how it works. Lie down and get comfortable. Then, starting with your feet, progressively tighten and relax each muscle in your body. ("Relax, toes...") It takes time to go all the way from your feet up to your head ("Relax, forehead... relax, scalp..."), but be patient and include every muscle. When you're done, you'll feel as though you just took a hot bath. You'll feel warm and relaxed—and so will your back.

TIPS FOR REDUCING STRESS

Reducing the amount of stress in your life doesn't have to be time-consuming or complicated. In fact, it can be as easy as picking up the phone and talking to a friend. Here are a few tried-and-true strategies for ironing out some of those mental wrinkles.

- Exercise regularly
- Enjoy a sauna, steam room, or whirlpool
- Get a massage
- Practice meditation or visualization
- Do t'ai chi or yoga
- Spend a little more time with your hobbies
- Turn on some music
- Lose yourself in a good movie

Visualization. This is actually just a fancy name for daydreaming—but with a healing twist. When you practice visualization, you completely focus your mind on a relaxing, pleasing mental image—a lovely landscape, for example, or a soothing swim in gentle surf. Don't let your mind wander. Focus all your attention on the image you've created. Smell the clean, tangy air. Feel the sand massaging your feet. Enjoy the caressing warmth of the sun on your face. The more deeply you "lose" yourself in the details of the scene, the farther behind you'll leave your daily cares.

Meditation. Meditation is hardly a new technique, but it's still considered one of the best ways to relax. As with progressive relaxation and visualization, the idea is to step aside from your daily stresses and to relax your muscles so that they're no longer causing you pain.

There are many different styles and variations of meditation. Traditionally, people have meditated by repeating a single word, called a mantra, over and over. It doesn't matter what word you choose. (A simple word such as "calm" or "peace" will do.) Silently repeating it over and over for 15 minutes or even longer can put you in a state of profound relaxation. Doing this on a regular basis is like taking a daily vacation. You'll feel more relaxed and fit—and so will your back.

SMOKING AND YOUR BACK

Cigarettes do more than damage your lungs and heart. When you smoke, cells throughout your body—including those in the spinal disks—do not get enough oxygen. Over time, the cells begin losing the ability to repair themselves, and the disks start to break down. This is why people who smoke are more likely to have back problems than those who don't.

Another problem with cigarettes is that the airways, in an attempt to clear out smoke and mucus, trigger coughing. Coughs put enormous pressure on already weakened spinal disks.

Quitting cigarettes isn't easy. If you have tried to quit but haven't quite been able to do it, take a few minutes to call the local branch of the American Cancer Society, American Lung Association, or American Heart Association. These organizations offer programs that have proven to be very effective in helping people quit.

Although stop-smoking classes and workshops have the most success, if you need extra help, your doctor may recommend that you try a stop-smoking aid such as nicotine patches or gum. Along with the classes, these products can give you enough support to kick the habit for good.

STANDING UP TO BACK PAIN

Your spine is surprisingly strong and stable—but only when it's balanced. When you stoop or slouch, your body's center of gravity shifts. Your muscles and ligaments, rather than merely helping you stand upright, begin struggling to keep you balanced. This can lead to painful strains and sprains of the ligaments and muscles in the back.

What's more, when you have poor posture, the weight of your body isn't evenly distributed among the vertebrae. As pressure on certain vertebrae increases, the nearby bones and cartilage can begin to wear. This in turn increases the pressure on sensitive spinal disks, which can lead to a herniated disk, along with sciatica and other nerve pain.

Poor posture can also cause permanent changes in the spine, including posture-bending conditions such as kyphosis and lordosis.

Practicing good posture can be critically important for preventing (and treating) back pain. And it's not hard to do. It doesn't mean standing at attention all the time. You don't have to give up your recliner and resign yourself to a lifetime of perching on straight-backed chairs—not entirely, anyway. What it does mean is making an effort to allow your spine to follow its natural S-shaped curve by walking and sitting the way nature intended.

Here's how to see where (and how) you stand. When you're undressed, stand sideways in front of a mirror. Your posture is good when you can visualize a straight line running all the way from your earlobe, down through the front of your shoulder and the center of your hip, back behind your knee cap and ending up just in front of your ankle bone. In addition, your chin should be parallel to the floor and not thrust outward.

Proper posture is important when you're sitting, too. You can do the same straight-line test while sitting in a chair, only the line will end at the center of your hip.

Your posture naturally changes a bit as you get older. So it's not uncommon for older folks to stoop a bit.

THE POWER OF GOOD POSTURE

One of the best ways to prevent back problems is to stand and sit in such a way that you maintain the spine's natural S-shaped curve. And the best way to do this is simply by maintaining proper posture. Here are a few ways to have picture-perfect posture all day long.

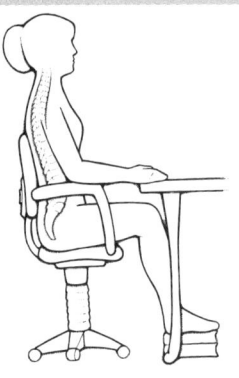

Sitting

Sit with your shoulders against the chair or couch back, with your chest lifted and your upper back straight. Your feet should comfortably touch the floor and your knees should be slightly above your hips (use a stool if needed). To keep your muscles relaxed, shift your weight occasionally—and get up to stretch every half hour or so. You may also find that a pillow or rolled-up towel behind your back will keep you comfortable.

Standing

Standing for a long time can be very tiring—and when you're tired you tend to slump. By distributing your weight correctly, however, you can relieve back fatigue and maintain good posture at the same time. The best way is to rest one foot on a raised object, such as a ledge, stool, or chair. This position bends the hips and knees and keeps your back from arching. Occasionally shift your weight from one leg to the other. Other helpful techniques include resting your hand or elbow on a ledge and standing with one foot in front of the other.

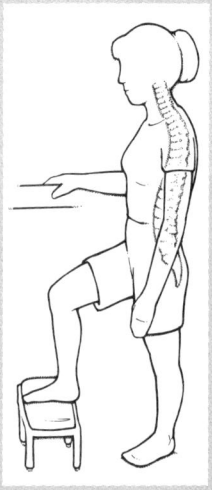

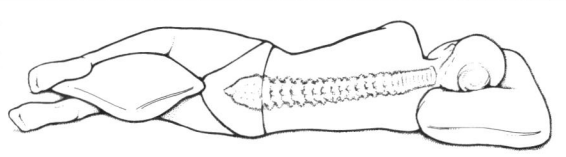

Lying Down

Sleeping on your side with your knees bent and a pillow between them is the best way to maintain the natural curve of your spine all night long. If you sleep on your back, place a pillow beneath your knees to prevent your lower back from arching too much. Sleeping on your stomach is the worst position for your back. But if you are only comfortable on your stomach, place a pillow beneath your belly to help keep your spine properly aligned.

Lifting

People often pick things up by bending over and using their back muscles to carry the load. This is extremely hard on the spine. A better way is to let your legs do the work. Face the object straight on, keep your back straight, and bend at your knees. Then stand up using the power of the large muscles in the legs, along with a little help from muscles in the back. Extending your neck backwards a lit-

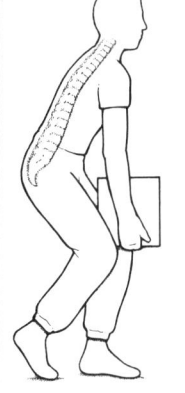

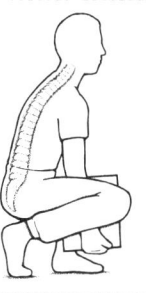

tle bit will also help you to maintain proper back posture as you lift.

When lifting, try to hold the object close to your body. Holding objects away from the spine while lifting can increase the load on the spine by as much as 15 times the original weight. And of course, if an object is unusually heavy, get some help. Your back will thank you for it.

By maintaining good posture when you're young, however, you can dramatically slow—and in some cases even stop—this process.

BACK CARE PRODUCTS: ARE THEY WORTH THE PRICE?

Along with fake diamonds and "ab"-strengthening devices, products for bad backs are hot items on the television merchandising circuit. Over the years manufacturers have introduced dozens of products—from "lumbar rolls" for back support to elaborate vibrating chairs—that are guaranteed (or your money back!) to take away back pain. But do they really work? And are they worth their sometimes hefty price tags?

Many of these products may, in fact, help ease minor back pain. Whether they're worth the cost is a question you'll have to decide for yourself. In many cases, doctors say, you can get the same relief without spending all the money.

Lumbar pillows. These tubelike pillows, which are shaped something like a Twinkie, are designed to give extra support to your lower back when you're sitting on the couch or in your car. Anything that supports the lower back can help ease back pain. But you can probably get the same benefits by slipping a rolled-up towel, or an ordinary bed pillow that's folded in half, behind your back.

The same goes for other "specialty" pillows, as well. The types of pillows that are marketed specifically for people with back pain are limited only by the manufacturers' imaginations. You can even buy an inflatable pillow that slips around your neck and is made for long-distance driving.

By all means, try them out. If you find one that seems to help, that's fine. But before you open your checkbook, spend a little time improvising. You may find that pillows you already have at home do just as good a job without the high price tag.

Vibrating chairs. If you have fond memories of Magic Fingers—those quarter-fed devices in motels that made the entire bed vibrate—you may decide that a vibrating chair is just the thing for back pain. There's no question that the soothing vibrations feel good and can ease muscle tension. But then again, so can a massage—and you can get quite a few massages for the cost of one of these chairs.

Specialty mattresses. A firm mattress is a necessity for people with bad backs. Mattresses that are too soft cause the back to sag, putting painful pressure on the muscles as well as the spine. Firm mattresses, however, conform to the natural curves of your back, providing solid support.

This doesn't mean you need to buy a specialty mattress made specifically for back pain. Although these mattresses may help, they're unlikely to be better than any other firm mattress. But they will be considerably more expensive.

If you're not ready to buy a new mattress just yet, here's an easy trick: Buy a sheet of plywood and slip it between the mattress and box spring.

The Balans chairs. Advertisements for Balans chairs say they are designed to ease back problems. Try one, and you may wonder what the fuss is about. As the chair has no back rest, you must continually use your trunk muscles to stabilize your body. And although the sloping seat does align the spine and evenly distribute weight, the chair actually feels less comfortable than ordinary chairs for most people.

To use the Balans chair, you must partly kneel on flexible knee pads, so your knees and lower legs bear most of the burden. Hence, many people find that sitting on the chair becomes painful after a while. Yet others say it helps relieve back pain. The only way to be sure is to try one for yourself. After all, your back is unique. It has its own shape and curves, and what works for one person may not work for you.

USING YOUR BACK WISELY

There's an arm of science that can give you a real pat on the back. Ergonomics is the scientific study of human work. It considers workers' physical and mental capabilities and limitations as they interact with tools, equipment, work methods, and the work environment as a whole.

What does this mean to you if your back hurts? One part of ergonomics is biomechanics—how your body moves as you go about your daily work activities. By studying how the different parts of the body move, scientists can make jobs and work places safer and more efficient. This not only increases workers' well-being but, along the way, reduces their back pain. And the principles of biomechanics can help your back at home, too.

The goal of biomechanics is to help you use your body in ways that maximize its natural strengths while minimizing stresses and strains. It's an important concept because how you move every day can have a major impact on your overall back health.

Unfortunately, this is one of the last things people think about. After all, it's easy to take a pill or to curl up in bed for a few quiet hours when your back hurts. But actually trying to change the many habitual ways in which you move— how you pick up a book, tie your shoes, put away groceries, or stand in line—takes a lot more thought and effort.

But it's worth doing. Your body moves thousands of times a day. Bending over once won't cause problems. But what about the 100th time—or the 10,000th? The strain adds up.

When a therapist or trainer teaches you the principles of biomechanics, you'll of course learn a lot about proper lifting. But biomechanics goes way beyond that. It can literally encompass every single move you make every day. Biomechanics means making sure that your desk is at a comfortable height. That your favorite chair is making your back better instead of worse. That your closet shelves are organized so that items you frequently use are within comfortable reach.

The goal of biomechanics is to shape and arrange your world so that you can move more easily and use your body in comfortable positions that don't put unnecessary stress on the vertebrae, disks, and spinal nerves. In the following pages, we'll look at some very practical—and very easy—ways to incorporate the principles of good biomechanics into your daily life.

Around the House and Yard

Think for a moment about the things you do at home. You're picking up children. Gardening. Taking out the trash. Vacuuming. There's a whole lot of moving going on. Here are a few ways to ease the strain.

Put up your foot. Standing with both feet flat on the floor is much harder on your back than standing with one foot propped up slightly. When you're standing for long periods of time, prop one foot on a low stool. If you're doing dishes, open the cabinet beneath the sink and stick one foot inside. This will reduce pressure on your lower back.

Support your arms. Whenever possible, use chairs with armrests. This allows your arms to assume some of the burden normally carried by the spine, which can help reduce back strain.

Shop for long handles. Whether you're buying a new rake or a new vacuum, look for a product with a long handle. The longer handle means you won't have to stoop, which is much easier on your back.

Use your legs. The muscles in your legs are much stronger than the muscles in your back. That's why doctors advise everyone—not just people with back problems—to always lift with their legs. It's a little awkward at first because it involves squatting rather than bending down to pick something up. But once it becomes a habit, you'll be amazed you ever did it any other way. We'll discuss proper lifting in more detail shortly, as it's crucial to back health.

Don't push yourself. This really has more to do with common sense than with ergonomics, but it's worth mentioning anyway. From time to time, we all get ambitious—or simply impatient—and work a lot harder than we should. This is especially true on weekends, when we're in a hurry to get our jobs done. The problem is that pushing tired muscles even harder invariably causes back pain—or worse. So do yourself a favor and punch the clock even before you think you've reached your limit.

Driving

Most of us spend a lot of time behind the wheel, and our backs pay the price. The truth is, most car seats simply aren't designed with the lower back in mind. What's more, the vibrations that occur during driving can be very hard on the spinal disks. To cruise in comfort, here are a few things to try.

Keep your knees high. To reduce pressure on your lower back, adjust the car seat so that your knees are slightly higher than your hips. Just make sure you can reach the brake without straining!

Move your hands. Periodically shifting the position of your hands on the steering wheel can significantly reduce the strain on muscles in your upper back.

Support your lower back. When driving long distances, place a small pillow or rolled-up towel behind your lower back. By supporting the spine, this can take a lot of pressure off the vulnerable spinal disks.

Take frequent stretch breaks. Getting out of the car and walking around now and then gives all your muscles, including those in your back, a chance to unwind.

Lifting

Unless you have a physically demanding job, you may not think that you do a lot of heavy lifting. But think again. Even folks who spend their days in offices are constantly bending down and picking things up. In some ways, your back doesn't care if you're picking up a paper clip or a 20-pound sack—though, of course, lifting more weight does cause additional strain. The mere motions of lifting can be very hard on the spine.

Studies have shown that people who lift objects improperly double their risk of a herniated disk, while those who do their lifting more carefully are much less likely to have problems. Here's how to do it right.

- Move in close to the item you're going to lift and spread your feet for good support.
- Bending your knees and keeping your back straight, lift the object, holding it close to your body. The farther away from your body it is, the more strain you put on your spine. A 10-pound weight held at arm's length actually puts a 150-pound load on your back.
- While lifting, concentrate on using your leg muscles. They're a lot stronger and more efficient at lifting than the muscles in your back.

What about back belts? In recent years, there has been a lot of controversy about the effectiveness of back belts in preventing lower back injuries. In a nutshell, the studies aren't conclusive. Although back belts do stabilize your back in side-to-side bending and twisting, they don't have the same effect when you are leaning forward to lift. Advocates of back belts argue that they remind wearers to lift properly and have reduced injuries in some workplaces (such as Home Depot, mentioned in chapter 4). However, chances are when workers are given back belts, they also receive biomechanics training, which could be a more likely explanation for improved injury rates. And some research suggests that belts may give workers a false sense of security, tempting them to lift even more heavy objects—which can increase their chances of hurting their backs.

Sex

This is one area in your life in which back problems can take a great toll—on your self-esteem as well as your pleasure. But a bad back doesn't have to mean a bad sex life. As with everything when it comes to sex, communication with your partner—about your need to protect your back as well as your relationship—is crucial. And if lovemaking is still difficult, be sure to talk to your doctor, too. Try not to be embarassed. Your doctor understands that your back trouble can affect this important part of your life, and he can provide specific information on the positions for lovemaking that are best for your particular condition.

Bear in mind that the basic rule for lovemaking that's loving to your back is: If it hurts, don't do it. This is particularly true when you've been having a flare-up of back pain. Even if you feel like making love—and chances are you won't just then—doing it when your back is already sore and inflamed is only going to make matters worse and slow your recovery time.

When you do feel ready to have sex, take a moment to give your back some extra support with pillows. One of the safest and most comfortable positions, for both the woman and the man, is to make love on your sides "spoon fashion," with the man lying behind the woman. In this position, both partners have their knees and hips bent, or flexed. They don't have to support their own weight or each other's.

Perhaps the best tip for back-friendly sex is to first gently rehearse sexual maneuvers by moving your body solo. Try moving as you would when you have sex to see whether your back is as ready as you are. This will show you clearly what your back can tolerate. Periodically, as your back pain improves and you'd like more variety, again practice a new position or motion by yourself before trying it with your partner.

Still need help? One excellent source of detailed information on making love with back problems is *Your Aching Back: A Doctor's Guide to Relief*, by Augustus A. White III, M.D. (Simon and Schuster Fireside, 1990).

Sitting

Have you ever wondered how many hours you spend sitting? Even if you're generally active, you can bet it's a lot—and sitting puts a lot of strain on the lower back. To reduce "sit strain," here are a few things you should do.

Get the right height. Unless you're tall, there's a good chance that many chairs are a little bit too high for you. Chairs that don't fit can be very hard on the back. (Here's a simple test: If you can't rest your feet flat on the floor without straining, the chair's too high.)

Add some extra support. Your lower back has a natural curve. Slipping a pillow or rolled-up towel between the back of the chair and that curve can take a lot of pressure off your lower back.

Sit up straight. Slouching down in your chair causes the curve in your lower back to slip forward, which can dramatically increase pressure on your lower back. You don't have to sit ramrod straight, but it is important to keep your lower back more or less flat against the back of the chair.

Raise your feet. It's helpful to raise your feet slightly when sitting, so your knees are at a level slightly higher than your hips. You don't need anything fancy. Simply resting one foot on a phone book will help reduce the strain on your back.

Move around. It sounds funny to say it, but sitting, from your back's point of view, is hard work. To give your back a break, periodically change positions—by crossing your legs, for example, or getting up and moving around for a few minutes.

Sleeping

If you're starting to think that dealing with back pain is nothing but work, here's a strategy you'll enjoy: sleeping. By making slight changes in your usual sleeping posture, you can help take some of the daily (or nightly) strain off your back.

The most back-friendly sleep position is lying on your side with your knees bent and a pillow tucked under or between your knees. Many people find those full-length body pillows a boon for this. Sleeping on your back is also good, especially if you put a pillow under your knees.

Sleeping on your stomach, however, is very hard on the back. But if you simply can't sleep any other way, you can reduce the strain by putting a pillow under your stomach. This will help maintain the usual curve in your back, so you don't wake up stiff and sore the next morning.

As we mentioned earlier, a firm mattress is a must because it helps support your back all night long.

Standing

Just standing still can be very hard on the lower back, which is why many people with back pain find they're actually more comfortable walking than they are standing around at parties or in line at the movies. If you want to reduce the strain of standing, here are a few things to try.

Put one foot forward. When you stand for more than a few minutes, it's a good idea to place one foot slightly in front of the other, which is less tiring for the lower back. Better still, rest one of your feet on a raised object, such as a step, rail, or footstool. This relaxes both your leg muscles and the muscles that support your spine.

Stand tall, not stiff. When you were a kid, every adult in your life probably told you to stand up straight and not slouch. It's true that standing straight is much better for your back than stooping or slouching. But don't take it to extremes. Assuming a military posture day in and day out will make your back hurt more, not less.

Sports

Back problems shouldn't leave you standing on the sidelines. Any exercise, including athletics, can be very good for your back—but only if you do it right.

Get some advice. Before starting a new sport, check with your doctor if you have a history of back problems. Some sports, such as bowling, can be very hard on your back, while swimming and bicycling are much easier—and, in fact, can usually reduce back pain. Other sports that can be hard on the back involve twisting (golf), rapid changes in movement (basketball), and repetitive impact (jogging on pavement). Simple changes such as learning to twist from the hips in golf, for example, or jogging on grass or on a low-impact indoor track, can make the difference.

In addition to talking with your doctor, don't hesitate to schedule an appointment with a tennis pro, a swim instructor, or whoever else is an expert in the sport you're interested in. Every coach has worked with people with bad backs and will be able to tell you how to enjoy the game without getting hurt.

Control your enthusiasm. It's one thing to be eager to start. It's another thing entirely to plunge into a new sport without giving your back—and the rest of your muscles and ligaments—time to adjust. Always take a few minutes to stretch and warm up before you start breaking a sweat. And if you're new to exercise, plan on taking it easy for the first several months or so. Going at it too fast too soon is almost guaranteed to stop you cold.

Travel

If you've ever found yourself heading to New York City while your luggage was en route to Los Angeles, you know that travel is one area in your life where you don't have a lot of control. But even when you're at the mercy of airports and impersonal hotel clerks, there are some very easy ways to protect your back when you're on the road.

Choose the right hotel. When making reservations, look for hotels that have gyms, heated pools, or whirlpools. Taking a few minutes to work out or simply soak in hot water after your flight will go a long way toward taking the kinks out of your back.

Pick a good seat. When booking your flight, request a bulkhead seat. These have considerably more legroom than other seats on the plane. And don't stay in your seat for long periods—get up frequently, move around, and stretch.

Pack lightly. The clothes you take are the clothes you have to carry. Do your back a favor by keeping the weight to a minimum. Before you start packing, think about shopping for a suitcase with wheels. When you're tired, your back is hurting, and all you want is to get home, you'll appreciate its "rollability."

Walking

Your body is designed to move, and walking is one of the best exercises for people with back pain. But don't make the common mistake of letting fashion take precedence over comfort and health. Unless you're walking only a very short distance, put on some running shoes or another comfortable style. Soft-heeled shoes will help to cushion your spine from the impact of walking.

If you're a woman, now's the time to select from the intelligent new shoe designs that make comfort and fit high priorities. And whether at the office or out on the town, you need to leave high heels to those without back problems. In your case, high fashion for the feet is frankly foolish, and you'll pay a high price in pain.

If your back pain gets worse instead of better when you're walking, check with your doctor. Many people's feet have imperfections that can throw off their balance and put pressure on their spines. Your doctor will be able to recommend a solution—which may be as simple as slipping padded inserts with proper supporting arches into your shoes. And occasionally, unequal leg lengths greater than one inch can aggravate a low back problem. This situation as well can be easily corrected with shoe inserts.

An Exercise Program for You

Every so often, fashion designers come out with new lines of clothes that define "the look" for the coming year. Almost overnight, it seems, every teenager in America is wearing the same clothes, shoes, and hairstyle. Yesterday's fashion *faux pas* becomes today's must-have.

We don't think of medical treatments as trendy—and they certainly don't change every season. But as doctors gain more information about particular conditions, previously accepted treatments fall by the wayside as other, more efficient strategies become the "standard of care."

The treatments for back pain have seen some rather stunning changes in the past few decades, most notably in the area of exercise. Twenty years ago, people with back pain were advised to take a few aspirin and then take to their beds. Most experts believed that prolonged bed rest—for days or even weeks at a time—would give muscles, ligaments, and nerves in the spine a chance to heal.

It would be an exaggeration to say that long-term bed rest has gone the way of seamed stockings. For some people, in fact, it's an essential part of their care. But for most people with back pain, exercise, not a week in bed, is the preferred method of treatment. This is true not only for minor strains and sprains but also for many more serious problems, including herniated disks, back spasms, and some types of nerve pain. Even people who have had surgery are often advised to get up and get moving as soon as they comfortably can.

Exercise helps relieve (and prevent) back pain in a number of different ways. For one thing, it helps to keep muscles strong and limber, which in turn helps reduce the strain on vertebrae and spinal disks. Regular exercise also increases the flow of blood, oxygen, and nutrients to the muscles, while at the same time it removes accumulated wastes, such as lactic acid. Some research suggests that many cases of back pain are due to nothing more complicated than underexercised (and undernourished) muscles.

Particularly for women, exercise—especially weight-bearing exercises such as walking and lifting weights—can protect backs by causing their bodies to store additional calcium in their bones. This can provide a hedge against osteoporosis, the bone-thinning disease that is the leading cause of vertebral fractures in older women.

In one study, women who had experienced bone loss and were having back pain were divided into two groups. Women in one group did regular walking, stretching, and other kinds of exercise, while those in the other group stayed sedentary. At the end of the year, the pain felt by the women in the exercise group was 70 percent less intense than the pain felt by the nonexercisers.

Exercise also helps your back in some less direct ways. People who don't exercise tend to put on extra weight, and this, of course, puts additional strain on the spine. Plus, people who exercise produce more of the natural "feel-good" chemicals called endorphins, which can help relieve stress and anxiety. And stress and anxiety, as we've seen, can play key roles in causing back pain.

The great thing about exercise is how little you have to do to get real benefits. Walking or swimming several times a week will provide a solid aerobic workout, increasing the flow of oxygen throughout your body. A few minutes of stretching each day will help keep the muscles loose and limber. A little weight lifting and a few abdominal exercises, such as crunches, can be a big help, too.

In the following pages, we'll discuss some of the best types of exercise for your back, as well as some of the worst. We'll also explain how to do exercises safely, so the good things you're trying to achieve don't backfire and wind up making your backache worse.

GETTING STARTED

Have you ever wondered how health clubs can sell a thousand memberships—most of them in January when people are fired up by New Year's resolutions—when they have room for only 200 members? The reason is simple. Even though exercise doesn't have to be difficult, getting started almost always is. When your body isn't used to it, exercise doesn't feel very good at first. You get tired easily. Your muscles get sore. And let's face it, you're probably busy all the time. Going to the gym or putting on your walking shoes isn't always a priority when you still have to get dinner on the table and all you really want to do is to relax in front of the TV.

But if you can force yourself to keep exercising for a few weeks, you'll be amazed by how much better you start to feel. Not only will you be less fatigued after exercising, you'll have more energy all day long. You'll make tremendous progress as your muscles quickly adapt to their new regimen. And in most cases, your back will feel a whole lot better after a few weeks.

As with so many things, moderation is the key. If you're recovering from a serious back problem or your muscles are simply out of shape, you need to start slowly—by walking around the block once or twice rather than jogging at the high school track or by swimming two or three days a week instead of five or six. Don't be in a hurry. Pushing your body too hard will make you sore, not strong. And as you already know, nothing is more discouraging than waking up one morning even more sore than you were before.

Doctors say it's fine to begin mild aerobic exercise, such as walking, swimming, or aerobic dance, even when your back is acting up. For a more vigorous workout, such as lifting weights or doing abdominal exercises, it's usually better to wait until the pain is gone. Give yourself a few weeks to recover. After that, you can start working out.

Here are a few additional tips for getting started.

Get a health check. Even though most back problems respond very well to exercise, some do not. And even when your back is strong, some types of exercise will do more harm than good. If you have a history of back pain, it's essential to check with your doctor or physical therapist. Likewise, if you haven't exercised for a while, have a serious health problem, obesity, or are over 35, you should visit your doctor before starting an exercise program.

Love what you do. Perhaps the main reason people often have a hard time exercising is that they're forcing themselves to do things they don't really enjoy. Yes, bicycling can be very good for you, and it's often recommended for people with bad backs. But if life on two wheels simply doesn't suit you, it's not a good exercise because you won't do it. The same is true of jogging. Some people love it while others loathe it. If you're in the latter category, don't let your friends or anyone else convince you to buy a pair of running shoes. You simply aren't going to stick with it.

On the other hand, maybe you love to walk—not for exercise, necessarily, but because you enjoy being outside and smelling the fresh air. Take advantage of it. Walking may not look as though it's as healthful as running, but researchers have found that it's just as good. Besides, if you like it, you'll do it. And that's essential for staying in shape.

Tour the health clubs. You certainly don't need to join a gym to stay in shape, but it's often a great way to begin. For one thing, virtually every health club has personal trainers on staff, who can help you design the plan that's best for you. What's more, many health clubs today are sleek emporiums with good equipment, fun music, exciting dance classes, and even amenities such as hot tubs, saunas, and juice bars. You may find you enjoy the energy you get from being around other people. And after a hard day at the office, an hour spent unwinding at the gym can easily become a labor of love. If cost is a concern, your local YMCA, YWCA, or community center can be an excellent option with most of the equipment but fewer frills.

Keep it convenient. When life's calendar is already full, setting aside several hours a week to exercise can seem like an unbelievable luxury. This is especially true if you belong to a health club that's all the way across town. The only way to stick with an exercise plan is to make it as convenient as possible. If there isn't a health club nearby, it may not be a bad idea to begin with a simpler activity that you can do anywhere, anytime, such as walking or bicycling. After all, what could be simpler than lacing on your sneakers and heading out the door?

Put it on your schedule. One reason it's often hard to stick with exercise is that it often feels like an add-on—an optional activity in an already busy day. That's why doctors recommend making exercise one of your "must-do" activities and doing it at the same times on a regular basis. Brushing your teeth isn't exactly fun, but you've conditioned yourself to do it at the same times every day—and when is the last time you told yourself you were too busy to brush your teeth? Making exercise a habit—doing it at the same times on the same days of the week—will help ensure that you keep it up.

Start early. Maybe you're not a morning person, in which case this tip isn't for you. But many doctors feel that morning is the best time to exercise. It gives your metabolism an early boost, which will give you lasting energy throughout the day. More importantly, things tend to come up during the day—unexpected meetings, for example, or simply an overload of stress—which can make it difficult to work out later on.

Start slowly. As we mentioned earlier, many good intentions get derailed when, instead of feeling better after exercising, you actually feel worse. The truth is, some people overdo it at first. You don't try to run the company your first day on the job, and you shouldn't try to be an athlete when you're just starting to get into shape. Studies show that people who start out exercising at a moderate, easy pace are twice as likely to continue with it as those who go all out too quickly.

Are you a walker? Start out by walking slowly and not too far. When that gets easy, pick up the pace a bit. Walk briskly and swing your arms. Do that for a few weeks. Then if the spirit moves you, go for a fast walk or an easy jog. Doing it slowly usually means you'll do it longer and that's what counts the most.

Warm up and cool down. Stretching is an important and frequently overlooked part of any exercise program. Even when you're doing light exercise, take a few minutes to warm up before you start. Put your arms over your head and give a good stretch. Flex your thighs, your hamstrings and calves, your shoulders. What you're doing is forcing extra blood into the muscle fibers, which helps prevent tendon damage or muscle strains. Warming up doesn't take much time and can save you a lot of back pain later on. Likewise, stretch again after you exercise. It will help to keep you limber. (We'll "prescribe" specific stretches shortly.)

THE BEST EXERCISES FOR BACK PAIN

You don't need a medical degree to know that some kinds of exercise—a rough game of soccer, for example, or spine-twisting contortions off the diving board—may not be particularly good for your back. The same is true of sit-ups and some other abdominal exercises. But even people who have had serious problems with their backs can do most kinds of exercise, as long as they get into shape slowly and work up to the stresses and strains.

It is important that your exercise program ultimately encourages you to work through the discomfort and increase your level of function. Studies have shown that people with chronic low back pain who exercise to a *goal* (length of time or number of exercises) generally do better than those who limit their efforts as soon as they start to feel uncomfortable.

Everyone is different, of course, so you should always check with your doctor before beginning new exercises. But for the most part, you won't have any problem doing aerobic and flexibility exercises, as well as strength training and other forms of weight-bearing exercise.

Aerobic Exercise

People often think of "aerobic exercise" and "aerobic dancing" as being the same thing. While the dancing you often see in gyms is one kind of aerobic exercise, it's by no means the only one. Brisk walking, bicycling, swimming—

each of these is an aerobic exercise. They're among the best things you can do for your back.

Aerobic exercise simply means that you're moving quickly and steadily and forcing your body—including the muscles in your back and the spinal disks—to consume more oxygen. Aerobic exercise helps condition tissues throughout your body and improves their ability to repair daily damage. It's also the best thing you can do to keep your heart and lungs healthy.

Aerobic exercise is also a superb strategy for losing weight, which, as we've seen, can help reduce the risk of a herniated disk or a fractured vertebra.

For simplicity and low cost, walking is one of the best aerobic activities you can do. It's considered low-impact, which means it puts very little pressure on the spinal disks. And it has the added advantage of being a weight-bearing as well as an aerobic exercise, so it can help keep your bones strong.

Even small amounts of aerobic exercise can be very good for your back. Doctors recommend working out aerobically for 20 minutes (or more) at a time, three to five days a week.

Weight-Bearing Exercise

Gravity is a wonderful thing. Not only does it prevent your morning newspaper from floating up to the ceiling, it also puts gentle, steady pressure on your joints, muscles, and ligaments. Too much pressure isn't good for your back. But when your muscles push against gravity, they get stronger and more flexible. At the same time, your bones retain more of their calcium, which makes them stronger.

Simply, any exercise that forces your body to work against gravity is a weight-bearing exercise. Walking is a weight-bearing exercise in which you're moving your own weight. Lifting weights, of course, is also a weight-bearing exercise.

WALK YOUR WAY TO FITNESS

No other exercise is as easy—or, many people find, as satisfying—as taking a long walk. Here are a few things you may want to do to get the most benefit as well as the most fun.

- Get a good pair of walking shoes—your feet and your back will appreciate it.
- Schedule your walks on your calendar. Go at the same times on the same days.
- To make the time go quickly, get a portable tape or CD player and listen to music or books-on-tape.
- Find a friend to walk with. You'll have a better time, and you'll also have someone to nudge you out the door when you're looking for an excuse to stay home. Or take Fido—he needs it, too.
- Always do some walking on your designated days, even if you don't want to go the whole distance.

People with a history of back problems are often nervous about lifting weights. Caution is certainly needed, along with careful instruction from a physical therapist or your doctor. But when you do it correctly, weight lifting can strengthen muscles throughout your body, making them better able to withstand (and reduce) the stresses on your spine.

If you belong to a gym, you'll have access to an exciting range of weight machines as well as free weights—all the barbells, dumbbells, and other weights you hoist without benefit of machinery. But you can also lift weights at home using nothing more complicated than a pair of 5- or 10-pound dumbbells—or even cans of food.

Begin with small weights and multiple repetitions, then add weight gradually over several weeks. You can also start by lifting from a lying position, which supports your back. And, you may find a back support belt makes lifting easier.

As far as your back and bones are concerned, it doesn't matter what kinds of weights you lift, as long as you do it carefully and regularly and you get good instruction before starting.

Swimming, incidentally, is a superb exercise because your entire body is supported by water, reducing the strain on your back. What's more, research has shown that swimming can increase the amount of bone in your back. Studies have shown, for example, that women who swim three times a week will have slight increases in bone density, while women who don't exercise regularly will actually lose bone. Another alternative for people with bad backs is a water aerobics class, where you exercise using the resistance of water, or even by simply walking in chest-deep water.

STRETCHING

One of the best things you can do for your back—and the one that often gets neglected in favor of other, more "exciting" exercises—is stretching. The benefits of stretching are subtle, so they're not always felt right away. But done regularly, stretching helps prepare the muscles for movement. Doing as little as five minutes of stretching a day can get rid of stiffness, strengthen the spine, and relieve painful compression of the vertebrae. In short, it's one of the best things you can do for relieving (and preventing) back pain.

It's almost impossible to hurt yourself by stretching. That said, it's still important to not overdo and to keep your range of motion within comfortable boundaries. If you feel pain while stretching, be sure to back off a bit.

Here are a few simple stretches that have been shown to be very good for the back.

Warm-up stretch. Lie on your back with a pillow under your head and one or two pillows under your knees. Simply lie still for 5, 10, or even 20 minutes. This is a very comfortable position that takes a lot of stress off your spine. You can do this as a warm-up before you start stretching or simply for relief during back pain flare-ups.

Single leg pull. Remove the pillows from under your knees. Place one small pillow under your head, so your spine remains properly aligned. Wrap your hands underneath your right knee and slowly pull it toward your chest. Hold for a count of five and release. Repeat with the left leg. Do the stretch three to five times with each leg.

Double leg pull. Place your hands under both knees and pull them together toward your chest. Hold for a count of five and release. Repeat three to five times.

Lower back rotation. Lie on your back with your knees together and slightly raised. Gently rotate your hips to one side while turning your head to the other side. Hold for a count of five and release. Then repeat, rotating your head and hips in the other direction. Repeat 8 to 10 times, alternating sides each time. (Avoid this exercise if your back is sore, however, as it may aggravate some low back pain.)

Leg pull-over. Lie on your back with your shoulders flat on the floor. With your left hand, gently grip your right knee and pull your right leg across your body toward your left side, turning your head in the opposite direction. Hold for a count of 10 and release. Repeat with the other leg. Repeat four to six times, alternating sides each time.

EXERCISING THE EASY WAY

It's easy to talk about exercise—but not so easy to do it and stick with it. Not only is time a factor, but not everyone enjoys sports or gym activities. But even if you hate the very idea of exercise, there are many ways to stay fit simply in the course of your daily routine. You won't even know you're exercising—but you'll still get the benefits. For example:

- When you go to work, park at the back of the parking lot, so you have to walk a little farther. Or get off the bus or subway one block early.
- Whenever possible, take the stairs instead of the elevator.
- Rather than having the newspaper delivered, walk to the nearest convenience store or "honor box."
- Take the battery out of the remote control. Simply changing channels by hand will help get you up and moving.

CROSS-TRAINING

In their own ways, aerobics, weight-bearing exercises, and stretching are all good for your back. To get the most benefit, however, you should combine all three. This is known as cross-training.

The advantage of cross-training is that it reaches every part of your body, from the muscles in your back to the heart muscle, from the ligaments in your thighs to the tendons in your back. Cross-training keeps you balanced, making each part of your body as strong and fit as the others.

This isn't to say that you need to do all three types of workouts every time you exercise. The principle behind cross-training is simply to alternate your workouts. For example, you might attend a yoga class on Monday, lift weights on Tuesday, and take a brisk walk on Wednesday. Or stretch for 15 minutes, then walk for 20 minutes. Or spend some time on the stair-climbing machine, followed by a swim. It's entirely up to you how you mix and match exercises. As long as you do all three, the benefits—more strength and flexibility and less pain—will make a real difference in how you feel.

EXERCISES YOU CAN DO AT HOME

Once you make the commitment to exercise and start following through, you'll quickly notice improvements in your energy and overall strength. You'll have less back pain than before, and you'll be less likely to have problems in the future. Even people with potentially serious back problems such as weak vertebrae, herniated spinal disks, or occasional sciatic nerve pain can experience dramatic improvements from exercise.

The following exercises will help you target key muscle groups—in your back and abdomen as well as in your legs, chest, and arms. You don't need weights to do them. You don't need to sign up at a gym or even put on a pair of athletic shoes. You can do each of these exercises at home, using nothing more than a mat (or a soft rug) to keep your back comfortable.

Plan on doing each of these exercises up to 5 times daily to start. As you become stronger, you'll find yourself naturally increasing the count to 10, 15, or more. Pay attention to your breathing. When doing each exercise, exhale during the movement that causes the most strain, and inhale when the exertion is lightest.

BUILDING A BETTER BACK

Pelvic tilt

This is among the easiest and most effective exercises for strengthening your lower back and abdomen. Lie on your back with your knees slightly bent. Tighten the muscles of your abdomen while at the same time pressing your lower back to the floor and slightly raising your hips. Hold for 10 seconds, then relax. Aim for 10 to 20 repetitions.

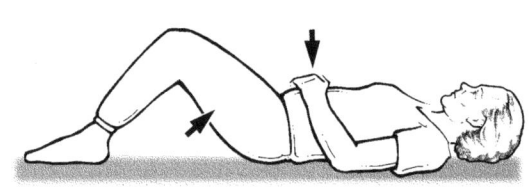

Modified crunch

The modern (and much safer) version of the sit-up, the modified crunch is the cornerstone of any abdominal work-out. Lie on your back with your knees bent. Holding your arms straight in front of you, slowly raise your shoulders a few inches off the floor. Hold for five seconds, then slowly lower your shoulders. Modified crunches can be hard at first, so don't be surprised if you can't do very many. Aim for 15 repetitions.

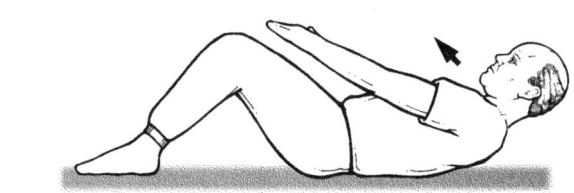

Crunch

This exercise provides a superb abdominal workout. Lie on your back with your toes hooked under the edge of a bed or couch, your knees slightly bent and your hands clasped behind your head or crossed over your chest. Slowly raise your shoulders and upper back off the floor, keeping your elbows parallel with your ears. Don't pull at your head—you want your abdomen, not your arms, to be doing the work. Hold for five seconds, then slowly lower yourself to

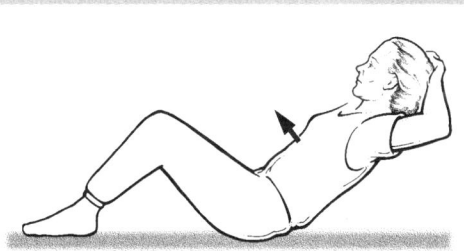

the floor. Try to repeat 15 times. If this exercise is diffi-cult, a pillow under your *upper* back and shoulders might help you get started.

Kneeling arm and leg reach

On your hands and knees, place your hands directly under your shoulders and about shoulder-width apart. Keeping your head down, slowly raise your right arm and left leg at the same time. Hold for five seconds, then relax and repeat on the other side. Continue alter-nating sides, doing five repetitions on each side.

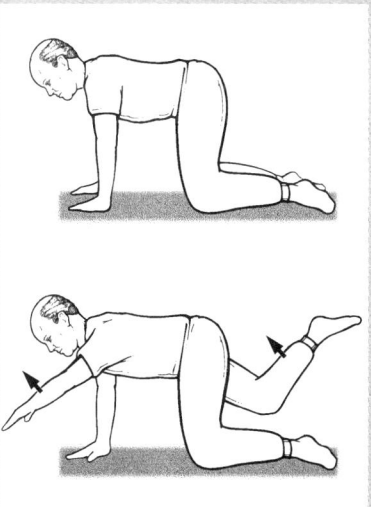

Modified push-up

This exercise targets primarily the muscles in your chest, arms, and abdomen. Lie on your stomach with your feet slightly off the floor and your hands underneath your shoulders, about shoulder-width apart. Keeping your back flat and your chin tucked in, slowly straighten your arms and push yourself up from the floor. Slowly lower yourself almost to the floor, then push up again. Try to repeat 15 times.

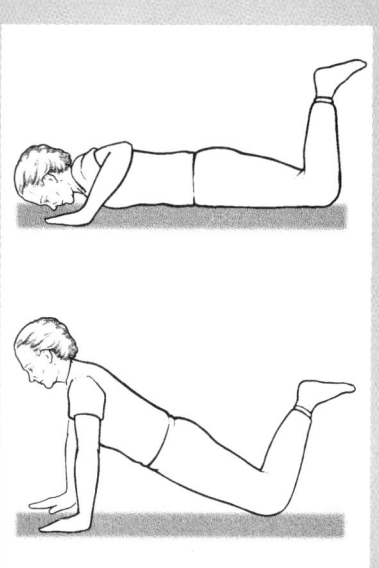

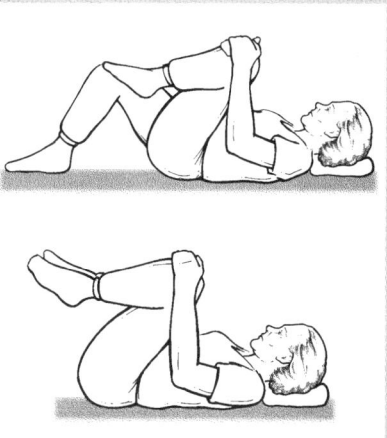

Knee-to-chest

Lie on your back with your knees slightly bent. Put your hands beneath one knee and slowly pull it toward your chest. Hold for 10 seconds, then relax and repeat with the other leg. Repeat five times. Then pull both knees toward your chest at once. Hold for 10 seconds, then relax. Repeat 10 times.

Cat stretch

This is a very popular yoga stretch for the lower back. Get on your hands and knees, with your hands directly beneath your shoulders. Slowly arch your back inward like a stretching cat, looking up as you do. Hold for a count of three. Then tuck your chin into your chest and round your back upward like a Halloween cat. Hold for another count of three, then relax. Repeat 10 times.

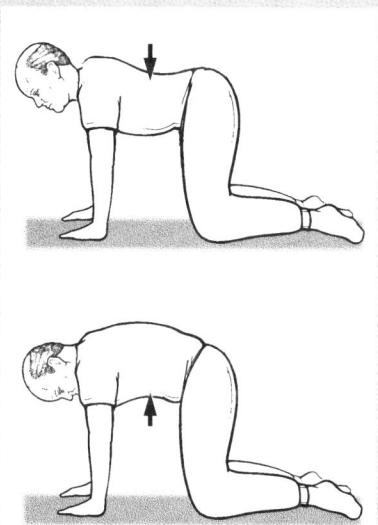

Fold-up stretch

This is another helpful exercise for the lower back. Get down on your knees and rest your buttocks on your heels. Stretch your arms out into the air in front of you, slowly lowering your chest forward as far as you comfortably can. Rest in the lowered position for a minute or two, breathing deeply.

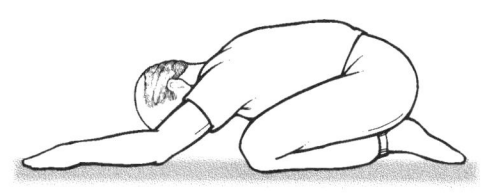

CHAPTER EIGHT

Complementary Care for Back Pain

Because back pain can be so overpowering at times, many people understandably strive for some sense of control over the problem—both for peace of mind and to promote healing. Some do this through faith, some through optimism, some by educating themselves about their backs, some with relaxation, some with exercise. While all these efforts are indeed helpful, what may make them seem especially significant is that they are things *you* control.

That same positive desire to pitch in and participate in your own back therapy can make you vulnerable to expensive and unproven remedies, however. Especially when your back pain keeps kicking up, it can be hard to resist the confident claims of many alternative therapies and products that simply don't work. At worst, some may harm you. Others may lift your spirits for a while or ease your pain momentarily.

If you want to pursue alternative treatments, two concepts are key: You don't want to hurt yourself or make your back worse, and you should never neglect or abandon standard medical care. You also don't want to throw away your money: Alternative treatments are seldom covered by health insurance. While there are many reputable alternative

163

practitioners, there are also many who are not—and who are all too willing to relieve you of your money for speculative treatments.

If you choose to visit an alternative therapist for your back, talk to your doctor first. Ask for recommendations, and be sure to ask about credentials and licensing. Bear in mind, however, that most alternative healers can hang out a shingle without extensive training, objective review boards, or any sort of consistent regulation. Unfortunately, it's often a case of "let the buyer beware."

With these warnings in mind, let's take a look at two types of alternative treatment that may have helped some people relieve some kinds of back pain. Unfortunately, as for most alternative therapies, there is little or no scientific evidence that proves these methods are helpful. However, some people do feel they have benefited by giving them a try.

ACUPUNCTURE AND ACUPRESSURE

We'll start with one alternative approach that does have some research behind it, although the studies are quite limited. Two of the oldest—and possibly most effective— complementary therapies are acupuncture and acupressure. According to the Food and Drug Administration, which regulates medical therapies, 9 to 12 million acupuncture treatments are performed in this country every year, at a cost of about $500 million. Many insurance companies, which are notoriously conservative, have begun to cover the costs.

Acupuncture and acupressure are ancient Chinese practices based on the theory that the body has a natural flow of energy called qi (pronounced "chi"). Qi flows through the body along 14 primary pathways known as meridians. According to Chinese practitioners, when qi gets blocked along one of these pathways, back pain (along with hundreds of other conditions) may result. Conversely, unblocking the channel can release the qi, giving relief.

So far, there is very little Western scientific understanding of traditional Eastern medical concepts such as qi and the meridian system. What research has been done centers on acupuncture's role in pain relief. Considerable evidence indicates that acupuncture may cause the release of pain-relieving chemicals called endorphins in the brain. The stimulation of acupuncture needles may also affect other body systems, including blood circulation and immune function, researchers say. One large study done in the 1970s, however, noted that for chronic lower back pain, acupuncture was of no statistical value.

When you see an acupuncturist, extremely fine needles are inserted into the skin. The needles stimulate key points along one or more energy pathways, removing blockages and allowing qi to flow freely.

Acupressure works in a similar way. Rather than using needles, however, the practitioner uses his hands to stimulate "pressure points" on the surface of the skin. Pressing on these points for three to five minutes, practitioners say, helps restore the flow of qi.

A Visit to the Acupuncturist

The practitioner will begin by taking a thorough medical history: When did your back problems begin? What activities cause the pain to flare up? Are you taking any drugs or undergoing other medical treatments? The practitioner will also ask you a lot of questions that don't appear to have anything to do with your back. As with most types of complementary care, acupuncturists and acupressurists take a holistic approach to healing. In other words, they believe that every aspect of your life—including things such as stress, emotions, and diet—can play a role in causing pain.

Next, you may be asked to partially disrobe and lie on a table. The practitioner will sterilize your skin with rubbing alcohol before inserting the needles into your skin.

Some needles will be placed in the area where you're feeling the pain. Others, however, will be inserted some distance away—in your arms and legs, for example. The principle of acupuncture is that back pain may be caused by blockages in one or more of your body's meridians. The blockages won't necessarily be located right where you feel the pain.

The needles may be left in place for 15 to 60 minutes. The practitioner may occasionally twirl the needles or pass heat or a low-voltage electric current through them to enhance the stimulation of the various pressure points.

If you've never had acupuncture, the idea of being a human pincushion can be unnerving. But the needles are exceedingly fine—some not much thicker than a hair. Most people say they feel only a slight tingling or ache when a needle is inserted. You may feel temporary heaviness in the muscle as well.

Is Acupuncture Safe?

The surgical steel needles used in acupuncture are sterile, individually wrapped, and disposable, so infection is extremely rare. Side effects aren't unheard of, but they're also rare. Certain acupuncture points may not be safe during pregnancy. Doctors have found that acupuncture treatments may stimulate the body's production of a hormone called oxytocin, which could cause premature labor.

To make sure you're getting the best and safest care, it's important to choose a practitioner who has the appropriate credentials. Acupuncturists are certified by the National Commission for the Certification of Acupuncture and Oriental Medicine, the American Association of Oriental

Medicine, the American Academy of Medical Acupuncture, and by many states. You can call any one of these organizations for a referral to a practitioner in your area.

MASSAGE THERAPY

The ultimate in hands-on care, massage increases blood flow to the muscles. Although there's no scientific proof, many practitioners also believe it delivers oxygen while removing waste products that cause pain, stiffness, and swelling. While the medical jury is still out on massage, you can certainly enjoy its enormously soothing and relaxing benefits, which make it a great strategy for easing stress and anxiety.

For a long time, massage was considered strictly an alternative therapy. Today, however, some doctors may recommend it for people with back pain. In fact, it's commonly used by physical therapists in back clinics and rehabilitation centers.

There are many different forms of massage. Some styles are quite vigorous and involve pressing and tapping on the back. Others, such as effleurage, are much more gentle. Regardless of the style, massage is thought to affect the nervous system by blocking pain signals from reaching the brain. It also reduces tension in the muscles, which is helpful for people with back pain.

Some people enjoy a massage once a week, while others make appointments only when their backs are acting up. If you've never had a massage, it's certainly worth a try. Massage is safe, although therapists usually recommend waiting a day or two if you've just strained or sprained your back.

Massage therapists are listed in the phone book. To make sure you're actually getting a therapeutic rather than an "adult" or sexually oriented massage, check to make sure that the therapist is licensed. You can call the American

Massage Therapy Association for a listing of therapists in your area.

THE 60-SECOND UN-WORKOUT

One of the most relaxing exercises that you can do—one that barely requires you to move a muscle—is called breathing. Don't laugh. Research has shown that deep breathing has a calming effect on the nervous system while at the same time causing a flood of oxygen to reach tissues throughout the body. This can go a long way toward relieving stress as well as back pain. In fact, many people say that after just one minute of deep breathing, they feel more energized, more productive, and pain-free.

Here's how to do it. While sitting or lying down, slowly take a deep breath. Fill your lungs until your chest cavity has expanded all the way. Hold the breath for a count of three, then exhale. Then simply relax for a minute. Let your mind wander as each breath passes in and out of your body.

That's all there is to it. Doing this just once a day will help erase stress, relax your muscles, and keep your back from throbbing. Best of all, it's quick, easy, and invisible, so you can do it anytime, anywhere.

Finally, whatever alternative treatment you choose, it's important that it be convenient and practical. The best (and cheapest) treatments are often those that you can do for yourself. You won't need to wait for a therapist's appointment, and that independence will foster a greater sense of control over your back pain.

CHAPTER NINE

New Strategies
for Back Pain

Many of us have fond memories of earlier, simpler times—when milk came in bottles and you could fill up your gas tank and still get change for a $10 bill.

People with back pain, of course, have less to feel nostalgic about. For a long time, surgery—along with bed rest and plenty of aspirin—was the only solution for many back problems. But times have changed—for the better.

As recently as 20 years ago, for example, people with herniated disks usually required major surgery—a lengthy incision followed by an even longer hospital stay. Today, as we've seen, most people with herniated disks don't go near an operating room. And even when surgery is required, the incision may not be much larger than the tip of a finger. Some people are even able to go home the same day.

Advances in the treatment of osteoporosis have been equally dramatic. Women in their later years are no longer advised to "take it easy" to protect the spine. Rather, they're encouraged to stay active, and to take medications when necessary, which can help strengthen older bones.

Treatments for virtually every type of back pain have undergone incredible advances in the past few years, and current research suggests that the future holds even greater promise. Diagnostic tests are getting faster and more efficient. Surgeons are pioneering new techniques that will be tomorrow's "standard of care." Even the psychological aspects, such as stress and people's individual reactions to pain, are likely to be on the forefront of back care.

In the following pages, we'll take a look at some of the most exciting new developments in recent years and where they're likely to lead in the future.

NEW HELP FOR OSTEOPOROSIS

Thankfully, the days are long gone when medicine responded to menopause as though it were a disease rather than a natural stage in life. Unfortunately, however, one of the hallmarks of menopause continues to be a serious problem.

When a woman reaches menopause, her body's production of estrogen begins to slow and eventually stops entirely. Low levels of estrogen cause the body's bones to begin giving up their calcium—and strength—at an alarmingly rapid pace. This condition, called osteoporosis, can be serious because as the bones get weaker, fractures of the spinal vertebrae—as well as of the wrists and hips—become increasingly common. (To assess your own likelihood of developing osteoporosis, see "Risk Factors for Osteoporosis" in chapter 2.)

Since osteoporosis is caused by flagging levels of estrogen, women past menopause are often given synthetic estrogen to boost their hormone supplies. Estrogen therapy is very effective at stopping bone loss and decreasing the risk of heart disease—but there may be a tradeoff. Some studies have shown that women who take estrogen for long periods of time have a higher risk of developing breast cancer (possibly amounting to an increased risk of 10 percent after 10 to 15 years of estrogen treatment). Other studies have indicated a possible increased risk of uterine cancer, but this is neutralized by the addition of a progestin to estrogen for women who take estrogen supplements alone.

Bone density measurements may help you decide whether to begin estrogen therapy. If you are a woman who has a personal or family history of breast cancer, you should discuss the risks and benefits of estrogen therapy with your doctor.

New Medicines, New Hopes

Estrogen is not the only medicine that has proven effective for osteoporosis. Two promising new prescription drugs, alendronate (Fosamax) and a nasal spray form of calcitonin, have joined the battle against bone loss.

These medications offer something estrogen doesn't. Not only do they help slow the rate at which the body loses bone, they actually help increase the density of bones that are already weak. This could have a significant impact on reducing the risk of vertebral fractures and other spinal problems.

Both medications work by affecting bone remodeling—the process by which the body breaks down old bone and replaces it with new. In our younger years, this process is essentially in equilibrium: New bone is created at about the same rate at which old bone is destroyed. When a woman reaches menopause, however, the balance takes a turn for the worse. As estrogen levels fall, the stimulus for bone cells to produce new bone is diminished. This is what causes bones to become fragile.

When women take alendronate or calcitonin, however, the process is reversed. The production of bone-destroying substances called osteoclasts decreases. This helps keep the bones strong, preventing fractures. The drugs aren't perfect, however, and doctors have been looking for ways to make them better. Let's take a look.

Alendronate

A new drug on the block, alendronate (Fosamax), recently has been approved for the treatment of osteoporosis. This powerful medication, which is taken orally, has been shown to slow bone loss as well as to help increase bone density—by 8 percent in the spine, 7 percent in the hips, and 2 percent overall. Although the percentages for bone growth alone are not huge, when you add in a nearly 50 percent decrease in vertebral fractures, the drug's potential is clear.

The problem with alendronate is that in a small number of people it may cause side effects, including muscle cramps, diarrhea, and a potentially serious irritation of the esophagus. But there are ways to reduce these problems and to make the drug even more effective.

- Taking alendronate first thing in the morning—or at least a half hour before eating—makes it easier for the body to absorb.
- Drinking water when taking the medication can reduce irritation to the esophagus. So can sitting or standing upright for a half hour after taking it.

Calcitonin

Calcitonin, a synthetic protein similar to a hormone produced by the thyroid gland, has also been shown to slow bone loss and increase bone density. It can be particularly helpful to people who are experiencing chronic pain from vertebral compression fractures.

Until recently, calcitonin was available only in an injectable form. That made it hard for people to use on their own. Now, however, it's available as a nasal spray, which makes it far easier to take. Calcitonin rarely causes side effects, although some people may develop nasal inflammation, a condition called rhinitis, or gastrointestinal problems such as nausea or loss of appetite.

(For more information on both alendronate and calcitonin, see "Drugs to Treat Osteoporosis" in chapter 2.)

Up and Coming

Researchers are investigating a number of new drugs that show great promise for treating osteoporosis in the future. It's too early to say for sure whether these drugs—which include a synthetic form of human growth hormone as well as new versions of vitamin D—will ultimately be successful. But researchers are optimistic that those new medicines may provide additional options for people who are trying to protect their bones.

One up-and-coming treatment, which is actually a new form of an old drug, has the most potential. For years, the mineral fluoride has been used to stimulate the growth of new bone. It works, but often causes nausea, vomiting, or diarrhea. Scientists have recently developed a version of the drug that is encased in a waxy coating. Instead of dissolving in the stomach, the new version travels intact to the small intestine, where it is absorbed. When this drug bypasses the stomach, researchers say, the side effects may pass you by as well.

NEW HOPE FOR PAGET'S DISEASE

Fortunately it's not common, but Paget's disease—a condition that causes bones in the spine and elsewhere to get thick and sometimes crumbly—can be extremely serious. In some cases, bones in the spine actually grow into the spinal canal, where they begin pressing on the spinal cord or nerves inside. And because it weakens the bones, Paget's disease can increase the risk of vertebral fractures.

Until recently, the only drugs that really helped were inconvenient to use or lost their effectiveness over time. They often caused side effects as well. In an exciting development, the Food and Drug Administration has approved alendronate (the same drug used for osteoporosis) for treating Paget's disease. This medication has been shown to help halt the growth of new bone that could threaten to invade the spinal canal. What's more, it helps make the bones a little bit stronger, so they're less likely to fracture.

ADVANCES IN SURGERY

Surgery for back problems has never been easy. As technology improves, however, surgeons are able to reduce both the amount of time people spend on the operating table and the discomfort they feel afterward. In addition, a few recent advances have made certain kinds of surgery much more effective.

Image-Guided Surgery

One promising though unperfected development is the use of image-guided surgery, in which a scanner takes moving pictures of the bones and cartilage during the operation. This can aid the surgeon in implanting devices. Unlike conventional X-rays or magnetic resonance imagining (MRI), this technology allows the surgeon to actually see how the spine moves and flexes while the surgery is underway.

So far, however, image-guided procedures are very expensive, and the scanner cannot exceed the accuracy of an experienced surgeon, doctors say.

Fusion Cage Surgery

One of the more difficult back operations is called spinal fusion. This procedure is sometimes necessary when more conservative treatment hasn't helped, when there is persistent pain from pressure on nerves or when a spinal deformity is developing. Bone (usually from the pelvis) is grafted between the vertebrae so that new bone will grow over it, fusing the vertebrae together and strengthening the spine.

A new type of device recently approved by the Food and Drug Administration may be helpful in certain spinal fusion procedures with very specific indications. Called an intervertebral fusion cage, the hollow device is filled with bone graft material and inserted between the vertebrae. The fusion cage supports the bones while the two vertebrae fuse together.

Although they do appear promising, fusion cages cannot yet be used in surgery for patients with osteoporosis, researchers say.

Percutaneous Vertebroplasty

As we've seen, fractured vertebrae are a leading cause of pain and disability among older women. There has never been an easy or effective way to repair a fractured vertebra, and the pain while waiting for one to heal can be excruciating. In fact, the only real solution—which wasn't always practical or effective—was to perform a spinal fusion.

But things may be about to change. Researchers at Johns Hopkins have pioneered a way to repair a damaged vertebra by injecting a tough glue, which holds the bone together. After the glue is injected, all the patient needs to do is remain still for several hours while the glue hardens. Once the fracture is "set" by the glue, pain can diminish rapidly or even disappear within hours.

So far, the procedure—called percutaneous vertebroplasty—seems very effective at strengthening bone. What's more, the procedure requires no incision. The glue is simply injected with a syringe through the back into the damaged vertebra. However, it is not yet appropriate for everyone, researchers say, and older vertebral compression fractures are less likely to respond.

COMING TO TERMS WITH STRESS

Doctors have known for a long time that stress plays a role both in causing back pain and in making the pain worse. It's only in recent years, however, that they've begun to realize how large a part stress actually plays.

In the past, people with back pain were rarely asked about their lifestyles or their jobs or whether they were happy or depressed. But this is going to change. Doctors in the future are certain to prescribe stress reduction strategies—such as meditation, exercise, and massage—just as often as they currently use medications and surgery.

EARLY ACTION

The scope of back problems—in terms of pain, disability, and costs to society as a whole—is enormous. It's significant to note that back pain is largely a Western problem, however. That may be because in developing countries, questions of basic health and survival are more pressing. It may also be because in our society, we generally live much more sedentary lives.

Regardless of the causes, researchers estimate that treating back pain in this country costs about $25 billion a year. When you add time off from work and lost productivity into the equation, the total may jump to $80 billion or more, and the economic toll is increasing all the time. Clearly, it's in all of our interests to do everything we can to prevent back pain in the first place.

One sensible approach to prevention might be to make "back school" a part of physical education in elementary grades. Childhood lessons in basic back ergonomics and how to prevent back injury might limit the flood of pain-plagued adults who enroll in therapeutic back school classes after the damage is done.

We also need to find ways to treat back pain more effectively, and researchers are starting to make this happen. As it turns out, one powerful solution that is emerging from research is actually the simplest. You can boil it down to two words: "Act fast."

At the first twinge of back pain, researchers say, people should take fast, positive action to prevent it from getting worse. In one study, a group of nurses—who have a very high risk of back pain due to the repeated bending and lifting required by their jobs—were given either physical or occupational therapy at the first sign of symptoms. Not surprisingly, they recovered much more quickly and with less pain than nurses who weren't given the "special" treatment.

The lesson couldn't be clearer. When your back starts acting up—whether from a day spent in the yard or from slipping on the stairs—and the pain doesn't settle down in seven to ten days, get help fast. Call your doctor. Get a massage. Do some stretching. Do anything, in fact, besides waiting to see if it gets worse. If you do wait, it almost certainly will. But even while it hurts, don't despair. Remember, most back pain will get better in 30 days or less.

FUTURE TRENDS

Although back pain often comes with aging and we can't always prevent it, we can learn to live with it more comfortably. Primarily, this will come through improved fitness, better diet, stopping smoking, learning to use our bodies in back-sparing ways, and becoming more aware of the dangers of back injury in occupations that require repetitive movements. Although back pain often makes people desperate for immediate relief, these practical approaches offer more hope than most alternative therapies such as acupuncture, researchers say.

While better education in lifestyle issues can help, there are also promising directions of study for medical science.

Future research into the physiology of pain, or how and where pain receptors in the body originate and how they chemically respond to pain, will lead us to better treatments. Once we know more about where pain begins, more effective medications will be developed. Likewise, more useful exercise programs, new nutritional strategies, and better education in body movement will also result from an increased scientific knowledge of pain.

And although some of the newest surgical devices are more effective than others, surgical inventions are promising. So far, techniques to reduce the invasive trauma and size of incisions involved in surgery, such as laser-guided procedures, haven't been particularly successful. But as the technology of surgical imaging continues to improve, these techniques will become much more effective. Soon, artificial spinal disks may be developed that will be implanted in the same way that joints such as hips and knees are replaced today. And looking a few decades ahead, spinal disk transplants from donors may also become commonplace.

As you can see, there is steady progress in back pain research. Fortunately, however, you don't have to wait for a bionic future to find relief. With the knowledge you have now, you have options. And with that knowledge, proper care, and a little luck, enduring endless back pain shouldn't be one of them.

APPENDIX 1
Suggested Reading

Managing Low Back Pain, W. H. Kirkaldy-Willis, Charles V. Burton, editors (Churchill Livingstone, 1992).

"Understanding Acute Low Back Problems," Consumer Version, Agency for Health Care Policy and Research. Call (800) 358-9295. (http://www.ahcpr.gov/consumer)

Your Aching Back: A Doctor's Guide to Relief, by Augustus A. White III, M.D. (Simon and Schuster Fireside, 1990)

Health Information Organizations and Support Groups

American Academy of Orthopaedic Surgeons
A professional organization that provides information about the prevention and detection of spinal problems.

> 6300 North River Road
> Rosemont, IL 60018-4262
> Phone: (800) 346-AAOS
> (708) 823-7186
> Fax: (847) 823-8125
> Internet: www.aaos.org

American Academy of Osteopathy
For a small fee, the academy will send you a list of certified osteopaths in your area.

> 3500 DePauw Boulevard, Suite 1080
> Indianapolis, IN 46268
> Phone: (317) 879-1881
> Fax: (317) 879-0563

American Chiropractic Association
Call for free publications about chiropractic care and back pain.

> 1701 Clarendon Boulevard
> Arlington, VA 22209

Phone: (800) 986-4636
           (703) 276-8800
Fax: (703) 243-2593

American Osteopathic Association
Call for free information about osteopathy.

142 East Ontario Street
Chicago, IL 60611
Phone: (800) 621-1773
           (312) 280-5800
Fax: (312) 202-8200
Internet: www.am-osteo-assn.org

Arthritis Foundation
Offers exercise classes and support groups in your area and provides free information about arthritis.

1314 Spring Street, NW
Atlanta, GA 30309
Phone: (800) 283-7800
           (404) 872-7100
Internet: www.arthritis.org

National Osteoporosis Foundation
A national volunteer agency committed to preventing osteoporosis. Call or write for free information about the diagnosis, treatment, and prevention of osteoporosis, or to find a bone-testing facility near you.

1150 17th Street, NW, Suite 500
Washington, DC 20036
Phone: (800) 464-6700
           (202) 223-2226
Fax: (202) 223-2237
Internet: www.nof.org

North American Spine Society
A national and international nonprofit association dedicated to spine care and spine research. Call for a list of physician referrals in your area.

6300 North River Road, Suite 500
Rosemont, IL 60018-4231
Phone: (847) 698-1630
Fax: (847) 823-8668

Osteoporosis and Related Bone Diseases National Resource Center (at the National Osteoporosis Foundation)
Provides information on the prevention, detection, and treatment of osteoporosis, Paget's disease, and other bone problems.

1150 17th Street, NW, Suite 500
Washington, DC 20036
Phone: (800) 624-BONE
             (202) 223-0334
Fax: (202) 223-2237
Internet: www.osteo.org

Spondylitis Association of America
A national nonprofit organization dedicated to educating the public about spondylitis and raising money for medical research.

P. O. Box 5872
Sherman Oaks, CA 91413
Phone: (800) 777-8189
             (818) 981-1616
Internet: www.spondylitis.org